Beat Fatigue
Handbook

By the same author:
Erica White's Beat Candida Cookbook

Beat Fatigue Handbook

Break free from chronic fatigue for good

Erica White

Thorsons

Thorsons
An Imprint of HarperCollins*Publishers*
77–85 Fulham Palace Road
Hammersmith, London W6 8JB

The Thorsons website address is www.thorsons.com

Published by Thorsons 2000

10 9 8 7 6 5 4 3 2 1

© Erica White 2000

Erica White asserts the moral right to
be identified as the author of this work

A catalogue record for this book is available
from the British Library

ISBN 0 00 710364 6

Printed by Omnia Books Ltd, Glasgow

Contents

Acknowledgements vii

Disclaimer ix

Dedication x

Foreword xi

Preface xii

Introduction: No Such Thing? 1

Part 1: Ten Pieces of Cargo 13

  1 An Invading Virus 15

  2 Allergy 21

  3 Nutritional deficiencies 33

  4 Toxicity and pollution 46

  5 Lifestyle 56

  6 Stress 62

  7 Hyperventilation 75

  8 Inefficient thyroid function 81

  9 Low blood sugar (hypoglycaemia) 87

10 Gut dysbiosis 94

Part 2: Beat Candida 109

11 Anti-Candida Four-Point Plan 111

    1 The Anti-Candida Diet 112

    2 Personal Supplement Programme 114

    3 Antifungal supplements 116

    4 Probiotics – the 'Good Guys' 120

    5 Support – the Fifth Point in the Four-Point Plan! 121

12 'Die-off!' 123

13 Some reasons for slow progress 127

14 The way ahead 131

Part 3: Feeling Great! 135

15 'Now I Feel Great!' 137

16 The author's own 'rags to riches' health story 153

Part 4: 'Let food be your medicine ...' 181

17 Anti-candida diet 183

18 Seven days' sample menus 189

19 Recipes for the sample menus 191

20 Guidelines for a General Healthy Diet 219

Part 5: Choose Life! 225

21 Nutrition: In Line with God 227

Appendix A: Candida score sheet 238

Appendix B: Useful Addresses 241

Appendix C: References and Recommended Reading 246

Index 249

Acknowledgements

First, I wish to thank those clients, past and present, who submitted their stories included in Chapter 15: 'Now I Feel Great!' They faithfully followed the advice which is outlined in this book, and have been rewarded with success stories to encourage fellow-sufferers from Chronic Fatigue Syndrome.

I also take this opportunity to express my heartfelt thanks to all my family for so lovingly 'putting up with Mummy' through all the years when I myself was ill. My fears that the children's memories of childhood would be marred by my constant sickness were unfounded; each one of them has developed into a caring and capable adult, a tremendous example of how all things can be turned to good! My heart is full of gratitude for the warm memories I have of my loving and supportive parents, and for my husband, Robin, who never once failed to be patient and understanding and who then gave up his own career to become totally involved in mine.

The friends now working with us provide loyal and enthusiastic support; I cannot adequately express the joy of working with a team which prays together! My thanks go to Pauline, Ann, Frances, Heather, Roger and Len. What would we do without you? I thank too those who are working with me as Associate Nutritionists under the Nutritionhelp umbrella, for their enthusiastic involvement: Heather, Ann, Fran, Marianne and Mary.

And as the work continues to expand, we pray for yet more labourers...

I am extremely grateful to Thorsons for giving me the opportunity to rewrite this book, previously self-published under the title *M.E.: Sailing Free*, so that they could produce it in this new expanded format and arrange for its world-wide distribution.

Some of the advice in the Action Plans appeared originally in factsheets produced by the Institute for Optimum Nutrition. It is very much adapted and extended, but I wish to acknowledge the source with gratitude, because most of my nutritional knowledge in any case was gained at ION through its excellent three-year course of study and subsequent postgraduate training. Thank you, ION; may you long continue to train many more practitioners in the field of clinical nutrition to meet the escalating demand for help from those who are suffering with chronic sickness due to nutritional ignorance.

Finally, I thank Patrick Holford, not only for once again agreeing to write the Foreword but for having the vision to set up the Institute for Optimum Nutrition in London right back in 1984, because this enabled me to become a Nutrition Consultant. I was extremely fortunate to have Patrick as my tutor, and I cannot thank him enough for inspiring me, for passing on some of his enormous enthusiasm and for having confidence in me.

Disclaimer: The author stresses that medical help and diagnosis should be sought before deciding to follow a nutritional regime specifically geared towards Chronic Fatigue Syndrome. In addition, this book is written in general terms and no responsibility can be accepted for individual situations where self-help is attempted without appropriate professional guidance. Although the author has done her best to ensure the accuracy of information in this book, she assumes no responsibility for errors, inaccuracies or omissions.

I dedicate this book to Robin –
my partner in marriage, work and life.

Foreword

by Patrick Holford, Founder of the Institute for Optimum Nutrition

Albert Einstein once said, 'The problems we have created cannot be solved at the same level of thinking we were at when we created them'. So-called CFS/ME is such a problem and, with old-style medical thinking, sufferers find themselves staggering around in ever-decreasing circles.

I am convinced that the 'Chronic Fatigue Syndrome' is the natural consequence for an individual living in an unnatural environment. By that I mean eating unnatural food, breathing polluted air, drinking polluted water and being exposed to unnaturally high levels of toxic bacteria, viruses and fungi, often as a consequence of an unhealthy digestive tract.

This new, enlarged and enriched edition of Erica White's excellent book presents a level of thinking applied to eliminate systematically the most commonly-found contributive factors which lead to chronic fatigue. Backed up by volumes of experience, most importantly her own, the information given is highly practical and proven to be effective.

Although necessary to change one's lifestyle, it is never easy but, with good support and management, I am sure that the vast majority of readers will benefit from following this advice and find themselves able to offload their unwanted cargo and sail free, back into a way of living which is in line with the natural design of the human body.   *Patrick Holford, 2000*

Preface

The **Introduction** of this book gives an overview of my understanding of the way in which the body's immune system becomes overloaded and unable to function efficiently, which I firmly believe should be regarded as the main cause of Chronic Fatigue Syndrome rather than putting the blame on an invading virus. 'Susceptibility' is the name of the game!

The 10 chapters contained in **Part One** discuss 10 possible contributing factors which increase susceptibility. The causes of each factor are considered, and advice given on what can be done, with the emphasis on a nutritional approach.

In **Part Two,** Chapter 11 contains a detailed explanation of the four-point plan that is needed to offload the last of the 10 factors discussed in Part One, a yeast called *Candida albicans* which has a strong tendency to overgrow in the intestines and invade the rest of the body. I have found this condition, to a greater or lesser extent, to be present in every single case of fatigue syndrome that I have come across, which is why I have devoted so much space to it. Chapters 12 and 13 discuss problems which might be encountered and some possible reasons for slow progress, and Chapter 14 explains the eventual way forward.

Part Three has two chapters. Chapter 15 contains personal testimonies from clients who have either successfully recovered from CFS (or are well on the way at the time of writing) by following the nutritional approaches outlined in this book and I very much hope that you will be encouraged by reading these real-life stories and first-hand accounts. I also hope that you will enjoy Chapter 16, because this contains my own story of 'sickness into health' and includes my discovery of several factors which had been placing loads on my immunity.

Part Four gives practical information and guidance about the anti-candida diet, together with a suggested menu plan for a week and all the necessary recipes to go with it, taken from my *Beat Candida Cookbook*. It also contains guidelines for a healthy diet once you are well, to show you what you are aiming for.

Parts One to Four stand complete if you are interested in discovering a nutritional approach to fighting Chronic Fatigue Syndrome. However, **Part Five** contains an 'optional' chapter which is included for those who are additionally interested in the role of nutrition in health from a Christian perspective. For me, this underlies all that I have learned and practise but I have no desire to force my views on those who do not wish to read them. However, to those of you who choose to read it, I pray you will be blessed and I guarantee you will be challenged!

At the end of the book you will find three appendices – a candida questionnaire so that you can assess the likelihood of yeast infection in your own situation, some useful addresses and information on how to find qualified nutritional help, and a reading list of books and journals that I have referred to in the text.

My hope for all who read this book is that you will be encouraged to look for and identify the pieces of baggage which are weighing you down and then discover how to throw them overboard. That way lies healing and health!

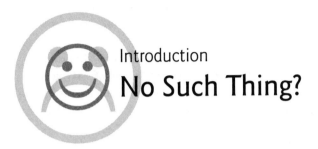

Introduction
No Such Thing?

By Any Other Name?

In writing about a health problem that is all too common, it helps if we decide right at the start what we're going to call it! 'Fatigue' is not enough, because the condition we are considering is fatigue of such severity that it is constant and unremitting, so it would seem to be a good idea to call it by the appropriately descriptive name of 'Chronic Fatigue Syndrome'.

In Britain, it is still widely referred to as ME (Myalgic Encephalomyelitis) though there is an increasing swing towards CFS. In America, there is the Chronic Fatigue Immune Dysfunction Association, so CFIDS is possibly the name best known on that side of the Atlantic – but can we agree that it's close enough to CFS for me to use it as a short-hand name through the course of this book? I hope so.

Not surprisingly, some of the names given to this illness are linked with epidemics so that it is sometimes known for instance as 'Royal Free Disease' because of an outbreak at the Royal Free Hospital in London in 1955 when 292 staff became ill together with a few patients. Unfortunately, the very bad press which has been given to CFS dates back to this time because two doctors were convinced it was caused by mass hysteria and refused to accredit it with the respectability of an acknowledged physical illness.

'Iceland Disease' is a name sometimes used because of an outbreak in that country in 1948, and in 1955, 500 were still experiencing chronic fatigue.

There was an epidemic in New York State in 1950 followed by a polio epidemic which earned it the name of 'Atypical poliomyelitis' and some years before that, in 1939, there was an outbreak in the Swiss army which was given the name 'Abortive poliomyelitis'.

Myalgic Encephalomyelitis translates into meaning inflammation of the brain, nerves and muscles, yet there is no consistent evidence of the swelling of the nervous system tissue which this name implies. Equally, Post-Viral Fatigue Syndrome is hardly an apt name if there was not an actual viral infection to start with – as can quite often be the case.

Of all the inappropriate names, 'Yuppie flu' is probably the hardest to accept or tolerate. CFS does not just happen to Yuppies (Young and Upwardly Mobile People – high-flyers and over-achievers) but to young children, elderly women and farm labourers! Neither is it just a form of flu, because influenza will normally go away in just a week or two. This name also manages to sound disparaging, suggesting that it is an illness which anyone could shake off if they really wanted to and it therefore carries an inbuilt accusation of malingering. We'll have none of that!

So, for the rest of this book, you and I will be speaking of CFS – Chronic Fatigue Syndrome – with all that the name implies.

Apart from epidemics, there have been countless individuals who suffered with this illness. From historical records, it seems probable that both Florence Nightingale and Charles Darwin had CFS. In recent times, another sufferer has been the Duchess of Kent. But you don't have to be royal or rich or famous to qualify – as possibly you can testify?

No Such Thing?

In the course of my work as a nutritionist, I have seen many clients express horror and disbelief when I have said that in my view there is no such thing as CFS! However, I hasten to put their minds at rest (and hopefully yours as well!) that I am not in the least suggesting that their symptoms are non-existent or simply 'all in the mind'. Far from it! As my own story later in this book will show, I know only too well the pain and misery of long-term sickness, and the frustration that comes from living with constant weakness and exhaustion.

So let me explain what I mean by this rather strong statement. In saying there is no such thing as CFS, I mean that it cannot be regarded as one specific illness with one specific cause, but rather it should be seen as a ragbag or conglomeration of many different conditions which vary from one sufferer to the next. Researchers around the world agree that the illness is made up of a combination of interacting factors so that there is no single cause – and therefore no single cure.

There can be no experts when it comes to dealing with CFS. The challenge for any practitioner is to discover and identify the specific set of problems affecting each individual sufferer. The most successful practitioners, whether medical or alternative, are those who are the best detectives!

A Ragbag of Problems

Recognizing the illness as a complex or ragbag of problems is very important. Let's say that a girl called Mary has been newly-diagnosed by her doctor as suffering from CFS, and she has a friend called Jim who also had CFS but has now got over it. Obviously, Mary will want to try the approach that worked so well for Jim. But Jim might have found tremendous benefit from having vitamin B_{12} or magnesium injections, and this does not necessarily mean that either of these will be helpful for Mary, in which case, if Mary's health fails to respond to B_{12} or magnesium, she will be disappointed and frustrated and even more in despair than she was before. The main causes of Mary's illness are obviously quite different from Jim's.

Many who have been formally diagnosed as suffering from CFS join a support group in the hope that they will benefit from communication with other sufferers and news of latest research, and there is no doubt that such contacts can be supportive. However, there are many who have never actually received a diagnosis, so they don't even have the comfort of knowing that there are countless others in the same boat; they feel very much on their own, often with little or no support from a puzzled or even sceptical doctor.

If a sufferer is branded a malingerer or hypochondriac, this creates an even heavier burden of loneliness, rejection and despair. In fact, it is estimated that in Britain alone at any one time there are around 150,000 people who suffer from CFS.

It is an illness which might have as many as 60 symptoms or even more. A client of mine once took the nutritional report I had prepared for her with my findings and recommendations, and showed it to her doctor. In it, I had carefully listed all the various symptoms she had reported in her questionnaire, but the doctor demanded, 'What is this woman saying? She says you have all these symptoms!' To which my client replied, 'No, Doctor, I told her all the things that were wrong with me; she hasn't made them up.' This lady said later that whenever she had reached the fourth symptom on her list, the doctor had just brushed it – and any other problems – aside. But, by its very nature, CFS brings with it a multitude of different symptoms for the sufferer to bear.

The first of the following two lists shows those symptoms which are most commonly associated with CFS, and the second is a longer list showing a wider range of symptoms, any or all of which (and more besides!) might occur in any particular case.

Symptoms most commonly associated with CFS

- Fatigue not relieved by rest; exhaustion after effort.
- Aches and pains all over, affecting both joints and muscles.
- Dizziness, poor concentration, poor memory, headaches.
- Nausea, wind, bloating, constipation, diarrhoea, irritable bowel.
- Over-reaction to heat or cold – shivering, sweating.
- Mood swings, anxiety, panic, crying, irritability, depression.

Symptoms which may be present

Muscle pain, muscle weakness, joint pain or swelling and stiffness, fatigue (physical and mental), drowsiness, lethargy, frequent infections of ears/nose/throat, sinusitis, rhinitis, asthma, eczema, acne, itching, sleep disorders, swollen glands, thrush, poor appetite, nausea, wind, bloating, constipation, diarrhoea, irritable bowel syndrome, cravings, water retention, loss of weight, weight gain, headaches, woolly head, lack of concentration, poor memory, anxiety, panic, crying, depression, irritability, mood swings, PMT, shivering, sweating, cystitis, palpitations, visual disturbances, sore eyes, dizziness, numbness, tingling, etc., etc., etc.

Possible Causes

So what are the causes of this ragbag of problems? I believe there are 10 major possible contributing factors and any of these, or any combination of them, might be overloading your immune system so that it is unable to fight and allow your body to become well. In fact, there is often a build-up of factors, each one of them paving the way for another until the total overload is just too much for the body to bear. Let me show you a typical chain of events, one which I see all too often in my work as a nutritional practitioner:

Frequent Chain of Events:

- Minor health problems over many years with poor diet, frequent antibiotics, the Pill or HRT, steroid treatments, leading to . . .
- Yeast in the intestines spreading and changing into an aggressive fungal form, leading to . . .
- Digestive and bowel symptoms, low energy, desire for more sugary foods and stimulants, leading to . . .
- Skin problems like acne, eczema and psoriasis, often more antibiotics or steroid creams, leading to . . .
- Menstrual and premenstrual problems, thrush, cystitis, allergies, often hormone treatment or more steroids, leading to . . .
- Extreme tiredness, mood swings, anxiety, panic attacks, irritability, aggression, depression. poor concentration, poor memory, migraines, insomnia, often pharmaceutical medication leading to increased liver toxicity, leading to . . .
- Worn-down immune system, constant infections, development of more allergies, chronic fatigue.

I wonder how much of that chain you are able to recognize in your own situation?

Yeast infection (candidiasis) has certainly been a factor in every single case of CFS that I have come across, to a greater or lesser extent – usually greater. In its role of weakening the immune system, candida can be seen as taking its place in a chain of events like the one just shown and can frequently be found in the history leading up to the time when CFS set in.

It would not be true to say that the cumulative effect of previous situations is always the case in CFS (at least, not apparently so), because sometimes a sufferer has fallen prey to a virus which seems to have hit him out of the blue. However, CFS does very often set in after a gradual build-up of events, and getting to the root of the problem is like taking layers off an onion as each successive situation is discovered and dealt with in turn. As I shall try to make clear, I strongly believe that the key to the cure of CFS lies in realizing that the main cause is not an invading virus but a person's susceptibility to that virus. A bug which threatens to overwhelm your immune system can only do as much harm as your immune system will allow!

An effective immune system would allow no house-room to an invading virus; the attempted attack would be thwarted, the virus would be controlled and ill-health would be avoided. The answer therefore lies in reducing susceptibility, and this can be done through taking the following steps:

1 Making changes in lifestyle and eating habits.
2 Correcting the balance of bacteria in the intestines.
3 Boosting the immune system and nutritional status with adequate supplementation.
4 Removing all identifiable loads from the immune system.

In these ways, the body can become strong enough to fight back and destroy any invader which has been able to penetrate its defences, whether it is a virus, fungus, allergen or some type of bacteria.

A nutritionist can help to unravel the complicated tangle of events and situations which together have caused CFS, but in the final analysis the responsibility for healing and for health lies with only one person – the sufferer! Some folk are just not prepared to do what it takes. They cannot really believe that the food they eat has anything to do with their poor state of health and they will not countenance the idea of giving up tea or coffee or chocolate or anything else which might be having an adverse effect on their bodies, even on a trial basis to see if it helps. They believe I am trying to deprive them of one of the only pleasures in life that they are still able to enjoy. This is understandable and of course they are free to choose, but they really need to consider that eating gives only a momentary pleasure, whereas the joy that comes with a healthy body will last for years!

Others may be willing to make drastic changes to their eating habits but there might still be stressful circumstances in their lives which are placing such a load on their immune systems that no amount of good nutritional advice will be able to restore their health. It is really important to find ways of dealing with stress, either by taking steps to sort out the underlying problems or else by finding ways of alleviating its effects – or even of rising above it! Help for this situation is discussed in Chapter 6 – 'Stress'.

I cannot leave this discussion of the emotional aspects of CFS without saying something about fear. It is not in the least surprising that someone with CFS should be full of anxiety about his health and his future, for so many aspects of life are affected – relationships, finances and career prospects, at the very least.

One way in which fear takes hold is over the question of exercise or activity. It is not unusual to receive a telephone call from someone who has been recovering well, saying, 'I overdid it yesterday, and I feel as though I have put myself back to square one. I won't do that again in a hurry!'.

A fear was implanted way back in their illness that CFS gets worse if you do too much, and now they have just proved it to themselves by going for a lovely walk, only to be full of aches and pains and nausea and exhaustion on the following day. Something needs to be explained and you will find more about it in Chapter 4 – 'Toxicity and Pollution'. It's to do with the fact that exercise stirs up toxins in the lymphatic system and tips them into the bloodstream. The point is that although this can be good and is in fact a necessary thing, the temporary symptoms it causes are unpleasant and can be frightening. However, if you understand what is happening, you do not have to live in dread of a relapse every time you feel like taking a walk. Of course, the amount of activity needs to be monitored so that the stirred-up toxins don't lead to too many unpleasant symptoms, but you need to realize that a certain amount of exercise is beneficial and will speed up the rate at which your body can offload toxins. Even someone who is very ill and bed-bound is well advised to do gentle assisted movements of arms and legs to aid in this process, and should not be afraid to do so.

Of course, I understand that for someone who has already made a big breakthrough in health and is almost completely well, it is obviously most distressing to feel suddenly as though they have taken a backward step. I well remember the lady who told me that she had been Scottish dancing for the first time in eight years, a joy she thought she would never again experience! Her delight knew no bounds – until the next day when she rang again to say how ill she felt and was afraid she had overdone it and brought on a relapse! I was able to reassure her that no doubt her lymphatic system had been working overtime due to all the unaccustomed activity of her muscles, and that almost certainly in a few days' time she would be feeling better than ever. She was!

Another aspect of fear is that it often seems to have become an integral part of the illness, so that eventually the sufferer is even afraid of becoming well again. After months and years of chronic illness, the possibility of a healthy future is often regarded not only with incredulity but also with a fair amount of trepidation. As a result, I often find people who are afraid to admit that they are now completely well, even when they quite obviously are! Sure enough, they had suffered from CFS for a long period of time, but now they are back at work and coping with home and family, experiencing no more tiredness at the end of a busy day than any other normally busy person. Yet they still hold on to the identity they have known for so long, still think of themselves as 'having CFS'. If, having fully recovered, they are determined to stick to a good nutritional programme for their ongoing health and approach me for a review consultation, they still write on their questionnaire that they suffer from CFS!

My job then is to assure them that no, they do not! They need to be encouraged to recognize and come to terms with how well they have become. It is a sort of identity crisis, and for some it can take a long time before they are ready to admit that they *used* to have CFS, but that now they are really well!

Sometimes I am asked to get involved at this level by praying that they will be set free from the fear that grips them. Other times I hear from an ex-client that they have realized for themselves how fearful they had become and, as a consequence, how much it had held them back from experiencing the joy that *should* have been theirs when their health and strength were restored. Having made this realization, they have then been able to make a determined effort to break free from the bondage of fear, with happy results!

It is a common occurrence, and one which I feel needs recognition and help more than is generally realized.

But people *do* break free and they *do* become completely well! I hope you will be encouraged to believe that it's possible for you, too, by the time you have read this book.

Possible Contributing Factors

I believe there are at least ten possible conditions which may be major causes of CFS, and it is quite amazing how the symptoms of each condition bear a remarkable resemblance to symptoms of the others. What is more, the problems typically associated with CFS itself would match an almost identical list under each of the 10 headings. Each one of the conditions places a heavy load upon the body's immune system, and together they have a cumulative effect which means that immunity becomes less and less effective.

I would like you to imagine that your immune system is a ship – the good ship *Immunity!* To start with, *Immunity* is sailing well, in spite of the fact that she is carrying a whole lot of cargo. But one day a torpedo hits her and makes a hole in her side, and then the effect of carrying so much cargo quickly becomes apparent! The combined weight of the loaded crates and boxes is enough to push the hole below the waterline, so that *Immunity* rapidly fills with water and will doubtless sink unless speedy action is taken to identify the heaviest pieces of cargo and throw them overboard. This will lighten the ship and enable the hole to stay above the waterline so that *Immunity* stays afloat!

For our purposes, the torpedo might well be a virus or it could be stress or any other factor which is known to damage the immune system. Equally, any of these situations might also be part of the cargo, creating unnecessary loads for the immune system to carry, so we shall look now at various factors which might be responsible. If specific burdens can be identified and removed – thrown overboard – this will enable the immune system to sail healthily on its way, undeterred by minor torpedoes which almost certainly will be shot at it from time to time!

So in Part One we shall be taking a closer look at 10 possible pieces of cargo, any or all of which might have led to a broken-down (or sinking!) immune system, and a diagnosis (whether actual or suspected) of CFS. They are:

1 Viral infection, past or present.
2 Allergy – food or environmental.
3 Nutritional deficiencies.
4 Toxicity and pollution.
5 Lifestyle – negative factors.
6 Stress, past or present.
7 Hyperventilation.
8 Underactive or inefficient thyroid function.
9 Low blood sugar – hypoglycaemia.
10 Gut dysbiosis – an imbalance of intestinal microbes.

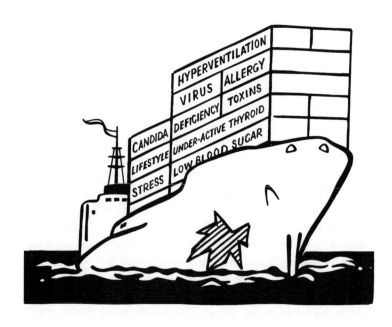

Part 1
Ten Pieces of Cargo

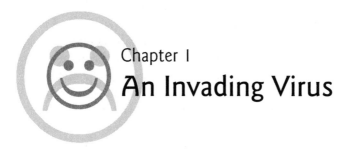

Chapter 1
An Invading Virus

Various types of virus have been implicated in cases of CFS. One is Coxsachie, of which several different types may be found within the gastro-intestinal tract, each of which also has a known tendency to affect muscle tissue. Coxsachie is extremely prevalent, and some researchers believe that it affects about 60 per cent of all CFS sufferers.

Another type is the Epstein-Barr virus which can cause symptoms characteristic of glandular fever (mononucleosis) and is a member of the herpes family. As you will know if you have ever suffered from cold sores (also caused by herpes), this virus has a habit of lying dormant and flaring up every now and then when the immune system is at a point of extra overload, which might account for the way in which symptoms of CFS sometimes ebb and flow. It tends to be found in adolescents.

The Cytomegalovirus is similar to Epstein-Barr but for some reason it mainly affects people who are past their teenage years, possibly in their 20s or early 30s.

Quite often, it is possible to trace the onset of CFS back to an infection caused by any of these viruses (in particular to glandular fever) or to influenza, chicken pox or German Measles (rubella) – or even to a vaccination against a common disease. In normal circumstances, our bodies deal with a virus by bringing into action various parts of the immune system to fight it, so if a viral infection hangs on and does not go away, as is often the case with CFS, it is obvious that for some reason the immune system is simply not up to doing its job. This might be due to one or more of the other pieces of cargo on board the good ship *Immunity*. A viral infection could be part of the overload of cargo; on the other hand, a virus might well have been the torpedo that made a hole in the side of the ship. In either case, *Immunity* is about to go under!

Jane Colby, writing in a journal called *What Doctors Don't Tell You* in December 1995, said that there was growing evidence to link CFS with polio. Back in 1948, when scientists first discovered the Coxsachie virus, they realized that although it was a very similar virus to the one which caused polio, its symptoms were actually different, so they named it 'Atypical polio'. This name was used again in the 1950 epidemic in New York State.

Jane Colby reported that recent advances in technology had placed the Coxsachie virus quite clearly in the polio family tree, so that CFS was sometimes diagnosed as 'non-paralytic polio'. Brain scans of CFS and polio sufferers showed very similar damage, or lesions. The overall similarities of the two conditions are not so surprising when it is realized that the viruses involved are members of the same family and use the same receptor sites in the body's tissues. Before the introduction of polio vaccines in 1954, outbreaks of CFS occurred immediately after outbreaks of polio in nine out of twelve cases, often involving hospital staff who had been caring for polio patients.

Obviously, the polio vaccine was a major breakthrough in terms of protection against a disease which had such devastating effects in terms of life-long paralysis. However, Jane Colby went on to say that, unfortunately, not all the effects of polio vaccination appear to have been good. Although the incidence of actual poliomyelitis fell quite dramatically, it seems to have opened up the way for an increase in other conditions, probably because the eradication of one type of enterovirus (gut virus) allows space for others to proliferate.

This seems to be clearly shown by the fact that, in 1959, the enterovirus which caused polio was responsible for 84 per cent of those paralysis cases which could be directly linked to an enterovirus. As vaccination against polio increased over the next two years, the incidence of polio-induced paralysis fell from 84 per cent to only 12 per cent but, during that same period of time, Coxsachie viruses increased to such an extent that by 1961 they were responsible for as many as 74 per cent of the paralysis cases that could be attributed to an enterovirus – not far short of the number previously caused by polio.

Yet in spite of these and other facts so clearly set out in *What Doctors Don't Tell You*, there are very many cases of CFS where no trace of a virus or of viral antibodies has been discovered so it cannot be assumed that a virus was a major cause of the illness in these particular instances.

On the other hand, and to confuse the picture even further, it is possible to find people who are carrying Epstein-Barr or Coxsachie antibodies who are not actually suffering from any signs of illness and in fact have never felt particularly unwell! To reinforce this point, the following interesting statement was made by Dr Thomas Stuttaford writing about polio in *The Times*, the British broadsheet newspaper:

… only a small number of those infected with the polio virus became paralysed; about ninety per cent didn't even realise that they had anything more threatening than a cold.

So what then is the deciding factor as to whether or not someone will develop CFS or polio or any other type of virus-induced condition?

Let me quote a final comment from Jane Colby:

> With polio and ME (CFS), *the state of your immune system governs whether you will be susceptible.* (Italics mine!)

This is an absolute reflection of my own strongly-held belief that a virus in itself does not have to be the cause of disease in our bodies; rather, it is the inability of our immune systems to fight against it. In other words, if the hole in the side of the ship is already close to the water-line, an added piece of cargo in the form of a virus will ensure that the ship goes down; but a strong ship that is not laden down with unnecessary cargo will be able to cope with that extra unexpected load – or even with a torpedo hole in her side – and still be able to stay afloat!

I'd like to make a few points for you to think about. Obviously, if you are invaded by a virus and you cannot shake it off, it is going to have an increasingly weakening effect on your immune system. In fact, some people are found to have excessive levels of interferon, which is our immune system's first line of defence against a virus. It is possible that this is an over-compensation for an otherwise weakened immune system but one of the effects of interferon is to make your muscles ache as happens when you have the flu. Perhaps you are one of those people who are suffering with CFS and who seldom catches a cold or flu, even when the rest of the family has them. If so, this is probably due to the fact that your immune system is producing high levels of interferon. However, as your health begins to improve and your immune system begins to get stronger, you may well then start to catch colds – which seems to be a contradiction in terms but actually means that your immune system has begun to wake up so that compensatory high levels of interferon are no longer needed. Of course, until you are fully well and your nutritional status is in top form, you are likely to be quite vulnerable because your immunity is still unbalanced and inadequate, but at least it's a step in the right direction.

If it is discovered that a virus is involved in a person's fatigue state, what needs to be questioned is whether the virus has *caused* the weakened immune system, as just discussed, or whether an immune system which has been weakened by *other* causes has allowed the virus to invade and take hold. Either way, I think you will agree that the answer *has* to lie in strengthening the immune system and to do this we need to refer to all the other pieces of cargo on the ship. Strengthened immunity can be achieved by improving nutritional status, balancing gut flora, dealing with the effects of stress, regulating thyroid function, controlling blood sugar, etc., etc. – in other words, by removing relevant pieces of cargo and lightening the load.

Let's be really clear about this. A virus is not the *cause* of a disease. It can only thrive and replicate and cause illness in your body if your immune system is unable to hold it back and control it, so we *have* to look at strengths and weaknesses of the immune system. I firmly believe that focusing on the virus has no future. The focus *must* be on reducing the susceptibility of the 'host' – the person in whom the virus is trying to take up residence or has successfully managed to do it – you!

There have been times in my life when I have had to endure several bouts of flu each winter, yet my husband didn't catch it once! There is no doubt that he inherited a much stronger immune system than I did, but also he carried none of the pieces of cargo which kept my immunity so low in the water and permanently ready to sink.

People who are carrying a virus like Coxsachie or Epstein-Barr yet display no symptoms at all of ill-health – let alone CFS – are obviously like my husband in that they have such strong immunity and are carrying so little unwanted cargo that the virus can make no impact on their bodies or their lives.

Another enigma often discovered in CFS is that even if there is clear antibody evidence of *earlier* viral infection, the virus is not necessarily still active, so why is the illness still persisting? For the answer to this, I believe we have to look at the other pieces of cargo which are weighing down immunity.

In his book, *Post-Viral Fatigue Syndrome*, Leon Chaitow says this:

> There is a viral connection with ME (CFS) in most cases, although we may never be sure whether this is the cause or a consequence of the process. Such ignorance, however, should not stop us from trying to eliminate the continuing viral drain on limited immune resources, while at the same time dealing with anything else which may be further reducing immune competence, such as stress and nutritional imbalances.

Here he mentions just two factors which are known to 'reduce immune competence', stress and nutritional imbalances, and both of these are included in my list of possible pieces of cargo, but as you now know there are also several others. Let's go on to look at them.

ACTION PLAN

1 Read the rest of this book!

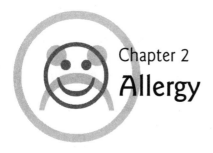

Chapter 2
Allergy

The term 'allergy' is one that is used by different people to mean different things! Probably the one point of agreement is that it should actually be reserved for a severe reaction to a substance leading to anaphylactic shock. Some people are affected in this way by peanuts or bee-stings, and they need urgent hospital treatment to reverse the effects and even save their lives.

More commonly, 'allergy' is used of situations like hayfever or asthma, where pollen or some other factor in the environment causes a reaction in those who have a sensitivity to it. Whether this should correctly be called 'allergy' or simply 'sensitivity' is irrelevant to the person who is suffering, but 'allergy' is the term they most often use.

When it comes to food allergy, there is the problem of whether it should more accurately be called an 'intolerance' or 'sensitivity'. I like the way Dr Jonathan Brostoff covers this predicament in his book entitled, *Food Allergy and Intolerance*. He quotes from Lewis Carroll's *Through the Looking Glass* where Humpty Dumpty says, 'When *I* use a word it means just what I choose it to mean...'. Dr Brostoff says that this sort of verbal anarchy should not be encouraged, but there is so little agreement over terms such as 'food allergy', 'food intolerance' and 'food sensitivity' (not to mention 'food idiosyncrasy', 'food hypersensitivity' and others) that anyone writing about this subject is forced to take Humpty Dumpty's line. There is no option but to select a set of suitable words and state clearly at the outset what you mean by them – which is precisely what I shall now do!

I find it necessary to make a distinction between those foods which cause an immune reaction and those which lead to an intestinal disturbance. I therefore use **'sensitivity'** when the immune system is involved, when for instance there are definite symptoms affecting the pulse rate, causing a headache or depression or making you feel *systemically* (by which I mean *all-over*) unwell. I use **'intolerance'** when there is no apparent immune reaction but a definite disturbance in the gastro-intestinal tract like diarrhoea, bloating or abdominal cramps, and I support the majority view that the only true use of the term **'food allergy'** is when anaphylactic shock occurs as a reaction to something like peanuts or crab.

Having said all this, the term most frequently used by the general public is simply 'allergy'. New clients will say to me, 'I know I'm allergic to dairy produce' or to wheat, or whatever it might be, so I tend to continue to communicate with them using the same language. In other words, I don't see why I can't take a leaf out of Humpty Dumpty's book and say that a word means just what I choose it to mean, providing of course I explain it.

It is really quite amazing how frequently I find that a CFS client is suffering (quite often without realizing it) from some type of 'allergy' (sensitivity, intolerance!), either to foods or to environmental factors, and sometimes to several of both types combined. The effects are not so severe that they are life-threatening, but the symptoms can be varied and severely incapacitating, affecting both body and mind with a list of symptoms that is strongly reminiscent of the list given in the Introduction of symptoms commonly associated with CFS. Apart from asthma, eczema and hayfever which most people recognize as having an allergic connection, symptoms can include sinusitis, brain-fag, fatigue, migraine, depression, panic, irritability, aggression, hyperactivity, hives, inflammation of the joints and muscles, bloating, swelling of the eyes and lips, rashes, constipation, diarrhoea and irritable bowel syndrome.

In my own story, I was virtually bed-bound with fatigue, weakness, aching muscles, woolly head, etc., for a whole year – until we eventually discovered that I was reacting to the then-new North Sea gas which had just been introduced to our area and piped into our house. Even before this, I was once rushed to the National Hospital for Nervous Diseases in London because my arms and legs had lost their feeling and were difficult to move. It transpired eventually that it was a severe reaction to some kind of spring-time pollen.

The increase in allergy has risen alarmingly in recent years. Official Government figures show that, since 1950, children in Britain are six times more likely to develop serious allergic disease, including asthma and eczema. Alexander Stalmatski, in his book *Freedom from Asthma* (1997), says, 'Surveys of UK schoolchildren conducted over the last ten years all point to the startling fact that in this country one child in eight now has asthma'. He says that these numbers have doubled in 20 years. Why should this be? The main reason, once again, is that the immune system is not working efficiently. So what is responsible for this trend?

One factor to consider is that this has been the era of antibiotics. It is assumed that such powerful drugs should enable us to live healthier lives and although they do indeed save life in many situations by killing invading bacteria, they also cause problems by destroying friendly bacteria in the intestines, allowing 'bad guys' to move in and causing an imbalance of gut flora *(see Chapter 10 – 'Gut Dysbiosis')*. The intestines then become permeable, creating a break-down of the boundary between the intestinal tract and the bloodstream. This means that toxins, bacteria and other unwanted rubbish can freely enter the blood from the gut, including incompletely-digested particles of food proteins which can leak through and then be regarded by the immune system as foes rather than friends, setting in motion a variety of possible reactions, none of them pleasant. The situation is known as 'leaky gut syndrome'.

Steroid drugs have also played a part because of their acknowledged immunosuppressant effect. Inhalers for asthma, creams for eczema and corticosteroid anti-inflammatory pills all have the effect of suppressing an appropriate and necessary response from the immune system. Such medications are now widely prescribed even for small children, and an increasing number of products are available over the counter without a doctor's prescription. In this category we also have to include any type of hormonal intervention, including the contraceptive pill and hormone replacement therapy, because both of these are actually forms of steroid treatment. If you want to intervene with the body's steroid hormones, you have to do it with other forms of steroid, but nobody ever tells a woman who takes the Pill or is prescribed HRT that she is actually having a form of steroid treatment. I have frequently seen women in their 50s and 60s with health problems caused by a broken-down immune system, including CFS, where the common denominator has been HRT. Some of them have been on it for a very long time, usually since having an early hysterectomy. Similarly, I have seen a tremendous number of women in their 20s and 30s with CFS who have been on the Pill for several years, sometimes since their early teens.

Immunization is a controversial possible explanation for the explosion in recent years of allergic symptoms in children. You just have to think about the onslaught in infancy, before the immune system is fully developed, of whole cocktails of viral and bacterial substances entering the bloodstream. Certainly, the risks of immunization have to be weighed very carefully by parents against the risks of not having protection against specific diseases, but it's a tricky decision and one on which I never advise because either way it could backfire! However, I do recommend that they read *The Vaccination Bible* published by the journal *What Doctors Don't Tell You*, so that they can make a more informed decision.

There is also the problem of immunizations for travel, which in some cases have been known to trigger CFS, and again *The Vaccination Bible* booklet is well worth studying. My own view is that I do not see the point of taking the risk of overloading my immune system unless it is absolutely compulsory to be immunized in order to enter a certain country. In many cases it is not compulsory but the majority of people still feel that they really need to have the protection it affords, and medical practitioners in general advise that you do. My thoughts are that if a country's authorities have left an open choice about it, there really cannot be too much danger of catching a particular disease, otherwise the immunization programme would have been compulsory, not optional. However, that is purely my own view and I have based my decision upon it. It is something which each one of us needs to consider and decide for ourselves.

Also contributing to weakened immunity is the fact that pollution has increased and at the same time there has been a steady decline in the quality of our food. Both these situations are discussed more fully in other chapters. In addition, the last 50 years have seen a general decline in breast-feeding. Bottle-fed babies don't receive the natural immunity they would receive from breast-milk (at least, from the breast-milk of a well-nourished mother), and in addition they are fed with formulae from cow's milk which has a very high tendency to cause allergic reactions. All these factors have played a part in the quite dramatic increase of allergic conditions like asthma, eczema and food sensitivities. And any such reaction will not only cause symptoms in its own right but will place a load on the immune system, an additional piece of cargo on board the good ship *Immunity*.

Let's take a look at food 'allergy'. In some cases it can be due to an enzyme deficiency. Certainly this is true of cow's milk products and gluten grains – wheat, oats, rye and barley. If your body isn't producing the enzymes needed to digest these particular foods, it is unlikely that it ever will. Fortunately, there are products available which can provide the enzymes so that if for instance you are unable to avoid a milk or wheat ingredient when eating out, you simply take a little capsule to provide the lacking enzyme and this protects you from an otherwise unpleasant reaction. For a dairy intolerance, the capsule should contain the enzymes lactase (to digest milk sugar), rennin, bromelain and papain (to digest milk protein), amylase (to digest starch) and lipase (to digest fat). Such a complex of milk-digesting enzymes addresses the whole spectrum of what is involved in milk digestion. For digesting gluten grains, you need a supplement which provides the enzyme gluten protease and also amylase. Your nutritionist or health-store assistant should be able to point you towards appropriate products.

However, as I have already mentioned, a great many food sensitivities are due to a leaky gut which allows minute particles of incompletely-digested protein to escape from the gastrointestinal tract into the bloodstream, where the immune system sees it as a foe rather than a friend, and triggers a reaction. The problem is that if you eat the food frequently you will usually mask a sensitivity to it, yet all the time it will be putting a load on your immune system.

Food sensitivity can often show itself as addiction. If you are unknowingly addicted to a food or drink (possibly tea, coffee, chocolate, alcohol, wheat or dairy produce, to name but a few possibilities) and have to go without it for a period of time, you begin to suffer from withdrawal symptoms. Of course, you don't realize what is happening but you might feel 'low' or tired or irritable or develop a headache. Because you don't feel too well, you reach for the very thing which you know from experience will give you a 'lift' – for a while, at any rate. It might be a cup of tea or coffee, a bar of chocolate or a biscuit, a hunk of bread and cheese or a glass of wine or beer; you will know your favourite 'pick-me-up'. Each time you do this you are feeding your addiction. Being addicted is a pretty good indication that you are in fact allergic (hypersensitive) to the very thing which you feel is doing you good, yet the 'lift' it gives is fooling you!

A craving for wheat or any other food or drink can be just as powerful as a craving for heroin. I once had as a client a beautiful 17-year-old girl who was suffering from bulimia. Her cravings and binges were so severe that her mother had to put padlocks at night on the food cupboards, refrigerator and freezer cabinet. One night, the girl crept downstairs and discovered some goods that had been forgotten and not unpacked. In the bag was a large packet of wheat flour – and she devoured the whole lot, straight from the pack! From this experience we were left in no doubt at all that she was allergic to wheat and that she was so addicted to it that this was the underlying cause of her powerful cravings and consequent binges.

There are of course all sorts of allergy tests available, but my own preferred method of testing foods is one which my clients can do for themselves and it costs them nothing at all! It's a pulse test. Decide first of all, by keeping a food-diary, which are the most frequently-eaten foods and consider them as suspects. By avoiding a food (or family of foods) for a minimum of five days, the immune system has time to forget how to tolerate it so that when the food is re-introduced you experience a more obvious reaction – either in terms of symptoms or by a change in pulse rate. It is usually one or the other. A significant change would be a rise *or* a fall of 10 beats or more per minute, but even a smaller change indicates that *something* is going on, and this helps to pinpoint a sensitivity. Digestive or bowel symptoms without a change in pulse rate, on the other hand, would indicate to me an *intolerance* to that food, rather than a *sensitivity* which would mean that the immune system had reacted to it. The Action Plan at the end of this chapter tells you how to do a pulse test.

Having discovered a food which is affecting your immune system, the obvious thing then is to avoid it until you can take steps to heal the leaky gut which has allowed it to develop. You will then hopefully find that the food may be re-introduced without difficulty at a later stage – often when candida overgrowths have been brought fully under control *(see Part Two – 'Beat Candida')*.

One interesting bonus attached to finding and then avoiding a problem food is that quite often it will lead to a very encouraging weight-loss. This is because the body can off-load fluid which had previously been stored in order to dilute the offending food and minimize its adverse effects – and fluid can be eliminated much faster than body-fat can be burned! However, the reverse is true if a gluten intolerance is found, because in this situation the walls of the intestines have been smoothed down and this drastically reduces the surface area through which nutrients can be absorbed. People with a severe gluten problem are suffering from coeliac disease and have to avoid gluten grains completely but others who have it in a less severe form suffer from a degree of malnutrition and consequent difficulty in gaining or maintaining weight. Discovering the problem and avoiding gluten grains can lead to a reversal of weight-loss, though often it doesn't start for a period of four to six months. Either way, if you have a problem with too much or too little weight, an intolerance or sensitivity to specific foods might well be the cause of it.

There is a very useful diagnostic urine test available from Great Smokies laboratory in North Carolina (practitioners in the UK have access through Health Interlink – *see Appendix B*) called the Intestinal Permeability Test. By drinking small amounts of lactulose and mannitol, the level of each of these two substances which has found its way into the urine shows whether or not the gut wall is leaky and, if so, to what extent.

Various factors help to cause a leaky gut and these include bowel disease (viruses, coeliac, Crohn's and ulcerative colitis all increase gut permeability), parasites, impaired digestion (insufficient secretion of digestive enzymes or stomach acid), medications (antibiotics, laxatives, chemotherapy, non-steroidal anti-inflammatory drugs including aspirin), refined foods, nutritional deficiencies, alcohol abuse, hot spices, detergents, the ageing process and physical trauma (surgery, radiation, burns, starvation).

In my experience it has been caused in nine out of ten cases by candida when it has burrowed through the wall, so that trying to heal a leaky gut while candida is still active is a bit like applying wood filler over woodworm holes if you haven't first destroyed the worms. They will simply pop up again round the edge! It is therefore important to do all you can to bring candida under control in the first place. In addition, the good nutritional programme involved in this process will provide nutrients like vitamin A, zinc and essential fatty acids which will all help to heal the intestinal wall so that sometimes, when you no longer have candida symptoms, you find also that the gut is no longer leaky and food sensitivities have disappeared. However, in many cases it is still necessary to improve matters and there are various helpful supplements which can be tried (see Action Plan), although this is one of the situations where you would almost certainly benefit from having professional advice from a nutritionist. When candida is no longer a problem, I have often known it take just a couple of months to heal the intestinal wall so that food sensitivities are overcome – although I have to say also that sometimes these problems can be particularly stubborn and take considerably longer to deal with.

Moving on to environmental sensitivities, these are often more difficult to trace than food allergies. I find it helps to run through a check-list of common culprits, because sometimes this will help to identify substances with which a client is in frequent contact and in this way it can help us to discover an unsuspected allergen. The list includes things like chemical smells, petrol fumes, animals, pollen, soaps and detergents, perfumes, plastics, pesticides, glue, varnish, paint and others. Mould is a common allergen, domestic gas is another. More often than you would perhaps suppose, I have to encourage my candida clients to find foster-homes for their house-plants so that they stop inhaling mould from the damp soil – and also more often than you would suppose, it makes an amazing difference to how they feel! Someone whose immune system has become hypersensitive to an overgrowth of yeast in their body will experience a reaction when they inhale (or eat!) moulds or yeasts which are related to the one in their body! Ridding the immune system of this and other burdens, including candida overgrowths, means that not only can you look forward to a reduction in food sensitivities but also to freedom from 'allergic' reactions to things you inhale.

Encouraging the client to do something about domestic gas will possibly involve them in a daunting and expensive process, but it can be positively life-changing, as I found in my own experience *(see Chapter 16)*. Drastic measures sometimes have to be taken. Meanwhile, if you realize or discover that you have a problem like this, do all you can to support your immune system with suitable supplements *(see Action Plan)*. You also need to support the liver in its role of detoxifying the body of pollutants *(see Chapter 4 – 'Toxicity and Pollution')*. Any or all of these factors might be implicated in environmental sensitivities. However, in due course, when your immune system has been strengthened, it should be able to cope once more with environmental loads, even if pollution and other pieces of cargo are still to some extent weighing down your immune ship.

In my own case I am now bothered by very few environmental substances, whereas for many years I experienced devastating reactions to springtime pollen, local anaesthetics, domestic gas, diesel fumes, paint and varnish. I still prefer to have low-odour paint when the house is redecorated, and not long ago I chose to go to another restaurant when the first one we walked into smelled strongly of new varnish – but that was simply because I saw no point in ruining the evening with an unpleasant smell (it still tends to linger in my nose), whereas once upon a time these factors created an utter nightmare in my life including a whole year of being virtually bed-bound because of North Sea gas!

ACTION PLAN

- **Change to a whole-food, healthy diet**, free of sugar, junk food, stimulants and chemical additives *(see Chapter 20 – 'Guidelines for a General Healthy Diet')*. If you are following the anti-candida diet *(Chapter 17)*, that's fine.

- **Take a good multivitamin and mineral supplement**, at the very least, to strengthen your immune system. Work out your optimum nutritional requirements from *The Optimum Nutrition Bible* by Patrick Holford, or consult a nutritionist for a tailor-made programme. Nutrients which have an antihistamine effect include vitamins C and B_5 and the amino acid L-Histidine. Antioxidants to help calm down free radical activity involved in allergic reactions include vitamins A, C, E, Beta carotene, selenium, lycopene and bilberry. It is possible to find all these in one combined supplement, or else you can take them individually.

- **If suffering from hayfever or asthma**, try taking 3000 mg of vitamin C up to four times daily (stop when it causes diarrhoea) and each time take 250 mg of vitamin B_5

(Pantothenic acid as calcium pantothenate or magnesium pantothenate) to a total of 1000 mg daily. Make sure you are also taking other vitamins and minerals as above.

- **Reduce or preferably avoid using bronchodilators** for asthma, rhinitis and sinusitis, and with your doctor's agreement try to reduce steroid inhalers (but only with his agreement). Also avoid steroid creams for eczema. Ask your nutritionist for alternative creams.

- **Learn about breathing techniques** for alleviating asthma, sinusitis and fatigue symptoms by reading *Breathing Free* by Teresa Hale. In many cases, simple breathing exercises can replace the need for a bronchodilator.

- **Use an alternative contraceptive to the Pill** and ask your doctor about stopping HRT; both of them are steroids and suppress immunity. There are in any case better ways of overcoming menopausal symptoms through nutrition.

- **Support your liver's detoxification processes** (*see Action Plan, Chapter 4 – 'Toxicity and Pollution'*).

- **Take all possible steps to bring candida overgrowths fully under control** (*see Chapter 11 – 'Anti-candida Four-Point Plan'*). After this, you can take specific supplements designed to heal a leaky gut. Try a supplement containing butyric acid or one containing L-Glutamine, N-Acetyl Glucosamine and Gamma Oryzanol, all known to be important to a healthy gut wall. In fact, the amino acid L-Glutamine taken on its own at higher levels is sometimes very effective. Many reputable food supplement companies supply suitable products for healing a leaky gut. Ask your nutritionist or health-store assistant for advice.

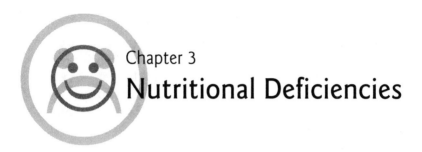

Chapter 3
Nutritional Deficiencies

I really want to impress upon you the fact that the role of optimum nutrition is absolutely fundamental to the efficiency of your immune system. Almost every family you can think of will have at least one member who is suffering from some sort of health problem, often of a mysterious and unaccountable nature. Many people react to various foods and chemicals, and some are allergic to almost everything. Our immune systems are finding it increasingly difficult to cope under the strain of all that is being thrown at them; our bodies were not designed to run on refined grains, added chemicals and polluted air.

So if you are suffering from CFS, it is impossible to over-emphasize the crucial role of taking levels of vitamins and minerals which are exactly right for you – as well as making any necessary changes to your diet.

Why has this situation of malnutrition come about when food is so plentiful in the Western world? In the last couple of centuries we have managed to turn our foods into substances which contain very few nutrients indeed. In fact, much of what we buy in shops under the guise of 'food' hardly deserves the name! Before the Industrial Revolution in 19th-century Britain, most people did not eat white flour, for instance. The invention of steel rollers in mills enabled manufacturers to refine the grain, removing its wheatgerm (the 'life') from the grain so that it would keep 'fresh' for a longer period of time without going bad. The general public welcomed this new product, believing it to be purer because it was white, and millers and retailers enjoyed the extra money they made from its longer shelf-life. But the parts of a food which go bad are the very parts which our bodies need, so food suppliers gain longer shelf-life at the expense of the public's well-being.

Sugar (in the form of sucrose) was once a very expensive commodity because it was taxed; when the tax was removed, sucrose became a useful ingredient to include in many products because of its preservative qualities, and again it did not take long for the general public to welcome these now widely-available sweetened food-stuffs and develop an increasingly 'sweet tooth', for which food manufacturers were more than happy to provide!

Until a couple of hundred years ago, the only sugar you would have consumed (unless you were very rich!) would have been fructose in fruit (and then only in season, unlike now when imported and frozen produce means it is freely available all year round) and honey (which you probably would not have eaten in excessive amounts). By the year 1900, you would have been eating some sucrose because it was cheaper by then, and the general level of consumption was about 4.5 kg (10 lb) per year. A hundred years later, the average Westerner eats more than his own body-weight of sugar every single year!

At the same time as sugar consumption began to increase, abattoirs made it possible for red meat and animal fat to become much more readily available. As the years went on, refrigerators and freezers made frequent meat consumption even more possible, and many people ate meat three times a day, all year round. Bacon or sausages for breakfast became quite normal, then ham or luncheon meat at midday, and a casserole or roast in the evening. More recently, the burger seems to have taken over at every meal!

In the First World War, the process of hydrogenation was developed. This process turns oils into spreadable margarines, and for the first time there was an alternative to butter or animal dripping. The consumption of margarine trebled in five years – and the incidence of heart disease rose with it. The reason for this is that adding hydrogen to natural unsaturated oils from seeds turns them from a healthy 'cis' form of fatty acid into an unhealthy 'trans' fatty acid, which has even more harmful effects than saturated fats from animal products. The chemical structures of the different types of fats show this quite clearly, but the consumer is generally either in a state of blissful ignorance or confused by clever advertising. Next time you buy margarine that is claimed to be high in polyunsaturates, look for the small print to see if it states 'hydrogenated'. If it does, put back the tub and look for one of the few which claim to be *un*hydrogenated – in other words, solidified by the less harmful process of emulsification. Your local health-food store should have a good selection of unhydrogenated margarines to choose from, made from different types of polyunsaturated oils including sunflower and soya bean. You will soon discover which is your favourite!

In addition to all the other changes in our food, manufacturers realized that chemical additives and preservatives could ensure greater profits, as did farmers using chemical fertilizers and pesticides on their crops, and hormones and antibiotics in their animal feed. We somehow forgot that food is the fuel for our body's machinery and that, unless the fuel is of sufficiently high quality and unadulterated, the machinery will start to run down and require an increasing amount of servicing just to keep it going. Besides having to cope with low-grade fuel, our bodies are infiltrated by an ever-increasing load of pollution from the environment. Small wonder that the machinery sometimes grinds to a premature halt!

The 20th century brought massive changes in our eating habits. Where we had previously eaten mainly vegetables and grains, we changed to a diet which contained as much as 60 per cent fats and sugars. We also changed to a more sedentary lifestyle – driving to work, sitting at desks all day, spending the evening watching television (having first spent some years listening in to the 'wireless!'), and buying our food in tins and packets instead of digging up the garden to grow it. We created a totally artificial energy balance, and our level of fitness deteriorated as a result.

As Third World countries latch on to our 'civilized' habits, their populations not only continue to suffer from deficiency diseases but also, increasingly, from Western diseases. Problems like heart disease and diabetes, once comparatively rare, now afflict the more Westernized sections of under-developed countries as much as our own. The situation is spreading.

Yet most of us consider that our dietary habits are 'normal'. If the truth be told, in the last couple of centuries we have completely forgotten what a normal diet is like and the vast majority of people are ignorant of what is happening. Like me a few years back, they have no idea of the connection between food and health. It is interesting how many of these same people insist on four-star petrol for their cars! However, public awareness is growing, and environmental issues form an increasing part of political policies. It is now recognized that lead from petrol exhaust has affected our children's learning and behaviour patterns. People are beginning to suspect that they might feel better if they knew more about which foods were good for them and which were bad. Migraines are commonly accepted to be triggered by chocolate, cheese or coffee. But do people realize that using refined white flour instead of wholemeal, for instance, increases problems with low blood sugar, causing first the symptoms of fatigue but then, if left unchecked, turning eventually into late-onset diabetes? That it also upsets the balance of essential minerals available to the body as well as its acid/alkali balance? And that its lack of fibre means it is one of the main causes of bowel diseases such as diverticulitis?

Do they realize it's their daily bread that might be making them ill? I once read that ducks on a pond had died when fed with scraps of white bread due to the bleach and chemicals it contained. I cannot vouch for that, but I can well believe it was true!

If, by some means or other, people do become aware of the situation, are they simply depressed or do they realize that there is in fact an answer, that it's *not* too late to improve matters, that something can still be done to ensure the health of our bodies even though we live in an unhealthy environment? The body has amazing recuperative powers if it is given the right fuel for its machinery.

Assuming that food is efficiently digested, it will largely be absorbed into the bloodstream as glucose from carbohydrates, amino acids from protein and essential fatty acids from oils. These are known as macronutrients. There will also be vitamins and minerals, known as micronutrients. There are many different nutrients in each category and they all have many jobs to do, both alone and in combination with each other. Without nutrients we would not be alive! The micronutrients (vitamins and minerals) are not able to provide us with energy, but on the other hand the macronutrients (carbohydrate, protein and essential fatty acids) cannot be used by the body without the aid of micronutrients.

Protein is needed by every single cell for all the processes involved in growth and repair. Consequently, if we are ill, it is vital that we eat good quality protein like poultry, fish, yoghurt, beans and pulses. Essential fatty acids, together with vitamins and minerals, are needed for healthy skin and hearts and for strong immune systems, and also to enable our hormones to work efficiently. If the nutritional status is good, there is no need for any woman to suffer the monthly miseries of premenstrual tension, or hot flushes at the menopause. Carbohydrate is needed for energy.

But although changing to a healthy diet is vital, food alone will not supply enough nutrients to repair exhausted glands, or ensure the right sort of cholesterol in the arteries once they have started to become blocked and hard, or restore an over-worked immune system. A careful programme of vitamins and minerals, at therapeutic levels, each in balance with its co-factor nutrients, is needed to undertake this kind of repair work. The damage caused to cells by dangerous free-radical molecules can be avoided if the right sort of nutrients, called antioxidants, are made available at adequate levels; research indicates that vitamins A, C and E and the mineral selenium all have effective antioxidant properties. For instance, taking good levels of vitamin C will help to counteract the harmful free-radical effects of passive smoking.

There is still a chance for our bodies to remain healthy, but we can no longer expect it to happen automatically. We need to know what to do, and then be prepared to make an effort to put our knowledge into practice. The medical profession has discovered a great deal which enables us to live longer lives than our forebears, but we ourselves must be the ones to take responsibility for the *quality* of this life we have been given.

The immune system is made up of many different parts which all depend on specific vitamins and minerals to do their work efficiently. For instance, there are two types of T cells known as Helpers and Suppressors, and these have to be in a proper ratio. The reason for this is that Helper cells stimulate B cells to make antibodies, whereas Suppressor cells appropriately oppose antibody production in order to keep antibodies in balance. If there are not enough Suppressor cells, stimulation by the Helper cells goes unopposed, leading to the production of too many antibodies by the B cells. Such a situation can lead to a heightened state of allergy and an increased susceptibility to auto-immune conditions, so the balance between Helpers and Suppressors is obviously crucial to health. And this balance is dependent on the body receiving adequate levels of vitamin A, folic acid and iron.

Particularly important for the immune system is vitamin C, and our requirement for this vitamin varies from day to day depending on what is happening in the body at any given time. If we are fighting an infection or an allergy, our bodies require far greater levels of vitamin C than when we are well, and it is a useful guide to take vitamin C to what is known as 'bowel tolerance' levels. This means that the body will take all the vitamin C it needs and, when it has enough, it will eliminate any surplus via the bowel and cause diarrhoea.

Leon Chaitow, in his book *Postviral Fatigue Syndrome*, speaks of the work of Dr Robert Cathcart, an American orthopaedic surgeon who is a strong proponent of using very high levels of vitamin C. Following the advice of double Nobel prize-winner Dr Linus Pauling, Dr Cathcart found that taking 15 grams daily of vitamin C cured his chronic allergy. Taking even more controlled a viral infection, and after that Dr Cathcart went on to evolve protocols for using vitamin C in the treatment of viral infections including hepatitis, and also reported remarkable results in treating people with AIDS.

Dr Linus Pauling, in an interview with Patrick Holford reported in the journal *Optimum Nutrition*, said, 'My suggestion is that every person who wants to have the best of health should increase the intake of vitamin C to somewhat less than the amount that causes significant looseness of bowel.' I have many times seen vitamin C when taken to bowel tolerance levels help to turn the tide in chronic illness, and it frequently avoids the need for antibiotics when a viral infection threatens to take hold.

It is a sad fact that our modern diet, made up as it is of many packaged and prepared foods, contains very little in the way of vitamins and minerals, even vitamin C. A lettuce once cut or pulled from the ground loses half its vitamin C content in half-an-hour, and I'm told you would have to eat 22 oranges to receive just one gram of vitamin C – but if the oranges have been picked when green and then allowed to ripen in a dark container ship, it is unlikely that they will have produced any vitamin C at all! What is more, drinks like tea and coffee actually deplete the body of vital minerals, as does sugar (sucrose), which might be called an 'anti-nutrient' because it supplies none of the nutrients required by the body and actually uses up important vitamins and minerals just to deal with it. More bad news comes from animal fat, which pulls against the benefits of healthy fatty acids found in unrefined seed oils and leads to wide-ranging problems from heart disease to premenstrual tension. Both sugar and fat have weakening effects on the immune system. No wonder our bodies have such an uphill struggle; it is amazing that we ever manage to hold our own against any invading bug! The role of optimum nutrition is absolutely crucial to health and, when there is repair work to be done, it is essential that you provide your body with the vitamins and minerals it is lacking in order to overcome and correct any biochemical deficiencies and imbalances which exist.

But if you are not a trained nutritionist, how is it possible to formulate a tailor-made programme of vitamins and minerals to meet your individual requirements? It can be done, and years ago I did it myself by poring over many books for weeks and months on end. However, this task is now made considerably easier by such books as *The Optimum Nutrition Bible* by Patrick Holford. In just 10 pages, Patrick gives a basic symptoms questionnaire and then explains how to convert the results into optimum daily requirements of each of the main vitamins and minerals. You then need to find appropriate supplements which will provide you with those levels as closely as possible. It's a good idea to fill in the questionnaire again after three months, because by then it is quite likely that your requirements will be lower. As an alternative to working it out yourself, of course, you can find a qualified nutritionist who will do the whole thing for you *(see Appendix B)*.

Discovering how to calculate optimum levels of nutrients when I trained at the London-based Institute for Optimum

Nutrition was, for me, like finding the missing piece of a jigsaw puzzle. I cannot stress too strongly that, unless the immune system is boosted by being given the right levels of the right kind of 'fuel' to repair the machinery and to help it run efficiently, you might just as well not bother with looking for ways to remove other loads from your immune system. It is as crucial and as basic as that!

Neither can I stress too strongly that each person's requirements are unique to them and to their present situation. For years now I have analysed several nutritional questionnaires every working day, and I am constantly struck by the fact that, although several clients might for instance be suffering from an overgrowth of candida and on the face of it have much the same collection of symptoms, yet their individual needs for vitamins and minerals will vary tremendously and will be unique to each person.

Clients often say to me that they have taken vitamins for years, to which my reply is that they cannot have done them much good, otherwise why do they need to consult me now? Often, when I look at the vitamin packet they bring to show me, I have to tell them that they have really been wasting their money because the levels of nutrients contained in the product are far below the client's actual requirements. Worse still, very often the supplements they have been taking contain yeast or lactose or other constituents which might have been making their particular problems even worse than they were before! It is worth remembering that B vitamins and certain minerals, for instance, are usually obtained from yeast so this will be the case with most multivitamin/mineral products unless it states clearly on the label that the product is yeast-free.

My experience is that if you get the supplement programme right and take these initial levels for the next three months, a review of the situation after that time will usually show that many of the symptoms have disappeared which means that levels of supplemented nutrients may be reduced accordingly.

Eventually, maintenance levels will be all that is needed to keep the immune system boosted and the body functioning efficiently, but this will usually take longer than three months to achieve so the situation needs to be monitored at regular intervals and the supplement programme updated appropriately along the way as health problems improve.

The philosophy that each one of us has an optimum daily requirement of nutrients is in total contrast to the idea behind the RDA (Recommended Daily Allowance) or RNI (Reference Nutrient Intake), a level which has been set by governments to indicate the average daily requirement of certain nutrients (not all – some are ignored) to prevent deficiency diseases within a population. The fact is that these figures vary from country to country, which seems rather strange, and they bear no relationship to biochemical individuality, neither do they take account of the therapeutic benefits of higher levels. Unfortunately, many people are misguidedly accepting the RDA (RNI) as being the only 'safe' level, above which anything else must be toxic, and so they are being deprived of the health-boosting benefits of realistic levels of vitamins and minerals to meet their own personal requirements.

My personal philosophy is that, even when we are completely well, we can only benefit from a small financial outlay spent on taking maintenance-level food supplements on a daily basis to help make up for the nutritional deficiencies in adulterated and depleted food. Apart from anything else, this will help our bodies to continue coping with the many varied effects of pollution. We have messed up our food and our environment to such an extent that our immune systems are in constant danger of breaking down under the load. However, I also believe that it is still possible to experience 100 per cent health if we are prepared to do something about it by eating as healthily as possible and by taking supplements to make up for the remaining deficiencies.

Once you are well, a good one-daily multivitamin and mineral complex will probably suffice, although you still need to take into account any special situations. For instance, if you have amalgam fillings they will constantly release mercury vapour so your body needs help to offload it by taking good levels of vitamin C, zinc and selenium. Another case for special consideration is a woman who has reached or passed the menopause, because she needs the right levels of magnesium, calcium (in a form which is well-absorbed such as citrate or succinate) and vitamin D in order to guard against the possible onset of osteoporosis. Meanwhile, until the day arrives when you just require a maintenance programme, let the therapeutic levels of vitamins and minerals you are taking do their work in helping you to achieve an optimum nutritional status.

It needs to be said that there are two situations which often prevent even the right levels of supplements from producing improvement. The first is poor digestion, which means that the body cannot absorb adequate nutrients, and the second is smoking because cigarettes will literally block the absorption of certain nutrients and destroy others before they have had a chance to do their work. Digestion and absorption can be helped by taking digestive enzymes and stimulating the production of gastric acids; the second situation really requires a determined decision to stop smoking – or at least to cut down drastically in the first place to fewer than five cigarettes per day. I have found that when I explain just how much of a part smoking is playing in their present ill-health, clients are far more motivated to stop than they are by thinking about the distant possibility of one day getting lung cancer. And good nutrition really helps in breaking an addiction.

I am constantly amazed at the appalling state of most people's nutritional status when they have their first consultation. Is it any wonder that their immune systems have crumbled? I hope that you are not one of these – but, even if you are, it's so easy to take steps to improve matters!

ACTION PLAN

1 Work out a tailor-made supplement programme to meet your optimum daily requirement of each of the main nutrients. See Patrick Holford's *Optimum Nutrition Bible* for how to do this.
   or
2 Find a qualified nutritionist to prepare a personal supplement programme for you.
   or
3 If you cannot manage to work out a tailor-made supplement programme for yourself and perhaps don't wish to consult a nutritionist, try to take the following levels of nutrients in a good multivitamin/mineral complex. If you cannot find them all in one product, or cannot find high enough levels, make up those that are lacking with additional suitable supplements.

Vitamin A	5000ius	Folic acid	200mcg
Beta carotene (natural)	5000ius	Biotin	100mcg
Vitamin C	2000mg	Calcium	300mg
Vitamin E	300ius	Magnesium	150mg
Vitamin B_1 (thiamine)	50mg	Iron	10mg
Vitamin B_2 (riboflavin)	50mg	Zinc	15mg
Vitamin B_3 (niacin)	75mg	Manganese	5mg
Vitamin B_6 (pyridoxine)	100mg	Selenium	100mcg
Vitamin B_{12}	10mcg	Chromium	50mcg

In addition, it's a good idea to take an essential fatty acid supplement. Unless you are advised to do otherwise, take a product which combines both GLA (as in Evening Primrose Oil) and EPA (as in fish oil or linseed oil, otherwise known as flax.) A basic level of each would be 150mg of GLA and 500mg of EPA/DHA. Essential fatty acids can also be derived from the diet

44

in seeds and their oils. (Recommendations based on *100% Health* by Patrick Holford.)

4 More specific advice on nutrient levels should be sought for pregnancy, menopause, children and athletes but the above levels are a basic guideline for an adult male or female.

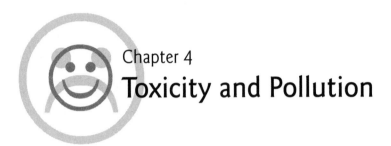

Chapter 4
Toxicity and Pollution

Toxicity simply means 'the state of being poisoned'! The body needs to defend itself against any form of toxin or poison which appears in the bloodstream, and so in situations of toxicity a tremendous strain is placed upon the resources of the immune system. For instance, if you happen to live near an oil refinery or in an industrial area, there is a good chance that exposure to its fumes will have helped to overload your immunity. We have lived for many years a few miles downstream of a refinery on the Thames Estuary, and when the wind is in the right direction, you certainly know it's there!

Some metals have a toxic effect on the body; these include lead (of which we received high levels from traffic exhaust before the advent of lead-free petrol), cadmium (from traffic but also from factory chimneys and smoke from cigarettes), aluminium (from toothpaste, indigestion tablets, deodorants, saucepans) and mercury (from amalgam fillings in our teeth). Some of these effects are now widely acknowledged. For instance, the British Medical Association has stated that aluminium plays a major part in Alzheimer's Disease or senile dementia, and high lead levels were shown to cause behaviour problems and learning difficulties in children who live in high risk areas of heavy traffic.

Even though the problems with lead have been reduced, we still continue to inhale cadmium from traffic fumes – and babies in buggies are just the right height to get it full blast.

Traces of mercury will be found in anyone who has amalgam fillings in their teeth. In Sweden, where it is recognised that mercury is the cause of many problems, it is now forbidden to give amalgam fillings to a pregnant woman because of the possible toxic effects on her unborn baby. In Britain, pregnant mothers are still encouraged to have their fillings free of charge, and you can be sure that most of these will be amalgam. Severe mercury poisoning is known to provoke symptoms exactly like those of Multiple Sclerosis. There is anecdotal evidence that people have recovered from CFS when their amalgam fillings have been replaced, but in my experience it is usually sufficient to detoxify the body of mercury by taking the correct amounts of appropriate vitamins and minerals, including good levels of selenium. Having the fillings drilled in order to remove them considerably stirs up their mercury content so that even if a responsible dentist takes precautions to prevent it, to some extent an even heavier load is placed upon the immune system and this can lead to a severe setback in symptoms. I can vouch for that from personal experience, because at one point my health problems were made considerably worse for a period of six months or so following the necessary repair of two crumbling amalgam fillings.

A hair mineral analysis can be very helpful for checking out the possibility of high levels of toxic elements such as mercury, lead or aluminium *(see Action Plan)*.

Other factors which produce toxicity are the many pollutants in our environment – in the air, earth, rivers, water-supply and sea, besides all the chemical additives and preservatives that enter our bodies with processed food and the cumulative toxic effect of pharmaceutical medications. All these factors are creating an enormous load for our immune systems to carry, and an already weakened immunity will simply not be able to cope. There have been reports that seals inhabiting the North Sea have died from viral infections. Viruses have been around for a very long time, so no doubt what has changed is the strength of the seals' immune systems which now work less efficiently because their food supply is contaminated with industrial pollutants.

I had a client in New Zealand who recovered well from CFS and returned to teaching a class of five-year-olds. She told me that in her class of 25 children, every single one had an asthma 'puffer'. We were having a long-distance telephone call and she could hear me gasp on the other side of the world! I said, 'But I thought you lived in a beautiful area, surrounded by fruit trees.' She replied, 'Yes we do, but the fruit trees are sprayed with pesticides.'

Some time afterwards, I reported this conversation to the father of a five-year-old girl in England. He was a visitor to our house and when he knew about my work he told me that his little daughter suffered from asthma and eczema. I told him about the class in New Zealand and he said, 'Oh, but it's just the same in my own daughter's class!' I know from statistics that asthma and eczema in children have escalated six times in the past 50 years, but I was amazed to hear first-hand that so many small children are now affected. If their immune systems are as weak as this at five years old, what on earth will they be like at 25? Unfortunately, steroid inhalers are now regularly prescribed and yet steroids are known to suppress the immune response – and in any case they do nothing about tackling the root cause of the asthma. Sometimes, just learning simple breathing techniques can bring about a dramatic reduction in the severity and frequency of asthma attacks *(see Chapter 7 – 'Hyperventilation')*.

Over the years I have collected some interesting facts about pollution, including the information that more than 28,000 tons of chemicals are used on produce by UK farmers every year, and that America exports 27 tons of pesticides every hour of every day. These facts alone raise some interesting questions. If the legal allowance of pesticides on produce is calculated on adult body-weight, what must be the concentrated effect in a child? And if crop-protection chemicals are formulated to stick and not wash off in the rain, how can we expect them to be washed off by tap water? In one year, the average person is thought to breathe in 2 grams of solid pollution and to eat 5 kg (2¼ pounds) of chemical food additives plus 4.5 litres (1 gallon) of pesticides!

Indoor pollution also needs to be recognized – vapour from synthetic materials in carpets and upholstery, insulation, cleaning materials, fumes from domestic gas, etc. Air conditioning makes matters worse by circulating the pollutants. A phenomenon has developed known as 'sick building syndrome', in which people working in a particular building feel ill all the time they are in it, obviously due to environmental factors. I have had three clients (a married couple and another lady) whose chronic fatigue was traced through hospital tests to carbon monoxide poisoning due to faulty gas fires in their homes. The lady was told by the hospital specialist that her toxic levels were so high she was lucky to still be alive. As soon as she gave me this information, I was able to formulate a specific supplement programme to help rid her body of carbon monoxide and its effects, and her health then started to improve – as happened with the couple also. The last I heard, they were going on holiday from England to America.

Lack of daylight can be counted as a form of indoor pollution because it leads to feelings of nervousness, exhaustion and irritability. It is important for people with a compromised immune system to receive at least two hours of daylight every day.

It is the liver which has the task of neutralizing all the toxins in the body, preparing them to be off-loaded via the kidneys, the bowel and the pores of the skin. Many people are walking around with toxic livers because they have taken large amounts of medicinal drugs over the years. Residues from these stay with us for a very long time. Then there are those who have a history of taking so-called recreational drugs, or of consuming high levels of alcohol; both these factors will leave the liver in a toxic state and put a long-term load on the immune system.

Toxins known as 'free radicals' are commonly found in food and in the environment as a product of combustion. We inhale them from chimney smoke, log fires, car exhausts and cigarette smoke but we also eat them with burnt toast and the crispy bits on roast potatoes! Seed oils like sunflower oil are extremely good for us if they are unrefined and not used for cooking at high temperatures, but once refined or heated as when frying chips, they are full of these dangerous molecules called free radicals. They attack us first of all by causing damage to a single cell in the body and then that cell, in an attempt to repair itself, takes a bit from its neighbour, thereby causing a chain reaction of damaged cells. Free radical activity is widely thought to be involved in allergy and in many other forms of illness including heart disease and cancer.

There is a lot we can do to reduce free radical attack, and obviously it makes sense to avoid cheap refined oils and burnt toast! It is perhaps even more important to ensure an adequate intake of the antioxidant nutrients which will 'defuse' free radical activity – vitamins A, C, E and the mineral selenium, sulphur-containing foods like onions and garlic, and certain amino acids including L-Glutathione and L-Methionine. Some very interesting research has also been done into the antioxidant properties of lycopene, a substance found in red fruits and vegetables, like tomatoes. In nature, as in seeds, nuts and grains, oil is always found with its own vitamin E content to help guard against free radical activity. However, the cheaper oils on supermarket shelves have had their vitamin E removed in the refining process – no doubt to be made into a supplement and sold as a separate item!

If you happen to be suffering from a leaky gut syndrome *(see Chapter 2 – 'Allergy')*, or if you have low levels of protective secretory antibodies lining your intestinal walls, toxins from the bowel will find it all too easy to invade the bloodstream, adding to the toxic load on the liver and immune system. Constipation should be avoided at all costs, because of the way it actually encourages the reabsorption of toxins back into the blood. Taking vitamin C to bowel tolerance levels is the best place to start, as already discussed in the last chapter. You can also take supplements providing appropriate fibre like psyllium husks, and sprinkle linseeds (flax seed) on to your breakfast and salads. Drink plenty of water.

On several occasions in London I have heard lectures given by world-renowned American nutritional biochemist, Dr Jeffrey Bland, who states that there is plenty of evidence to show that a toxic liver plays a major part in chronic fatigue, and also in multiple allergies. In my own experience, I have known many people whose health has started to improve – sometimes quite significantly – when appropriate nutritional steps have been taken to support the detoxification processes in the liver. One young mother, with a little girl and an 18-month-old toddler, had been ill for some time and completely lacking in physical strength since the birth of her second baby. After two months of taking some simple liver-supporting herbal supplements, she rang me to say that for the past week she had been pushing the baby's buggy the half-mile distance to and from her little girl's school, the first time she had been able to do it since the baby had been born. Although she was still not fully well, this increase in strength was an enormous encouragement to her. Another client, a girl of 19, had been bed-bound with chronic fatigue for the past two years, and her hands had contracted into the shape of a claw. When I suspected that she was in a highly toxic state and recommended a nutritional approach to help her liver work more efficiently, within a very few weeks she rang me herself to say that she was downstairs and dressed for the first time in over two years!

So what was the magic bullet I gave them? In fact, there is no single approach because situations vary so much, and the advice given to each of these clients had been different. We have to start with the understanding that the liver, apart from having a great many other significant roles, is central to the process of detoxification which takes place in two distinct stages, known as Phase I and Phase II. Phase I takes toxins from the blood and activates them, which means that they are altered in such a way that carrier molecules in Phase II are able to transport them out of the body. Phase I is like putting your rubbish into a sack in readiness for the bin-men to collect it and take it away, which is what happens in Phase II. However, all the various factors which increase the toxic load, including long-term sickness with its attendant long-term medication, has frequently led to a situation where Phase II is exhausted. This gives rise to a situation where there is a build-up of toxins as they enter Phase I but no way for them to be transported out of the body. Toxins therefore continue to increase, piling up behind the log-jam. This situation is particularly relevant in dealing with candida because of the large number of toxins it releases in its active state, and the even greater of number of toxins which invade the body when candida is destroyed. Phase II can often be overwhelmed. Fortunately, specific nutrients are known to stimulate Phase II and so can help to break the vicious cycle, and a diagnostic test (using urine and saliva specimens) is available from Great Smokies laboratory in North Carolina, USA, which can help to confirm and clarify the situation. This test is available to UK practitioners through Health Interlink *(see Appendix B)*.

Although you can take many simple steps yourself to help detoxify your body and support the liver in its work *(see following Action Plan),* where the situation is severe and chronic you really do need help from a qualified nutritionist who can arrange the test for you and then interpret the laboratory's findings and formulate a suitable programme to deal with the situations which have been revealed. Sometimes you might need to take an amino acid called L-Glutathione, sometimes you might need the help of certain forms of sulphur, sometimes you might need a combination of many things to encourage your Phase II pathways to get back into action. Sometimes it is Phase I which is shown to need attention because overactivity at this stage leads to an increase in free radical effects. Whatever you need to do, don't hesitate, because so often a back-log of toxins in the liver proves to have been a cork in the bottle as far as experiencing improvements in health is concerned.

I'd like to repeat the word of warning that I gave in the Introduction about what can happen when you start to feel better and become a little more active. At this stage, clients often ring me up and tell me that although they felt much better at the weekend and were able to go for a little walk, they obviously overdid it and now they are having a relapse. I quickly reassure them that this is not the case, and explain that the unaccustomed exercise, however slight, has stirred up some toxins in their lymphatic system, the drainage system that runs all around our bodies. The toxins which collect in this drain have to find their way eventually into the bloodstream so that they can be worked on by the liver and, as the lymphatic system has no pump, it is only the movement of our muscles which pushes the toxins around. Even the muscular movements involved in breathing will encourage toxins to circulate to a very small extent, but the movement involved in walking and swinging your arms makes an excellent pump, so that toxins are pushed into the bloodstream where they make you feel thoroughly ill. If your liver's detoxification processes are not efficient, the toxins will stay in the blood for a longer time than is comfortable, giving rise to aches and pains in the muscles, headaches, nausea, woolly-headedness and other general feelings of malaise.

This situation needs to be recognized for what it is so that you don't go into a panic about having a relapse and so that you take steps to improve your liver function. Exercise, when you can manage it, need not be avoided because of this experience, but you should certainly learn how to monitor the amount that you do by watching for the effects on the following day – until of course you have no more back-log of toxins to be taken into account!

ACTION PLAN

- Drink plenty of water – preferably filtered, otherwise bottled.

- Eat a healthy diet, with as much organic food as possible.

- Take vitamin C to bowel-tolerance levels – in other words, until you experience a slightly loose bowel motion each day – but make sure it's backed up by a comprehensive vitamin/mineral programme as discussed in Chapter 3.

- Particularly make sure that your multivitamin/mineral supplement contains good levels of the antioxidant vitamins A, C, E and the minerals selenium, calcium and zinc.

- Avoid constipation at all costs. If you can't face yet more vitamin C to take you to bowel-tolerance levels, try linseed sprinkled on your breakfast or your salad to help provide suitable roughage, and psyllium husks in supplement form will help to increase the bulkiness of the stool.

- Drink plenty of 'coffee' made from dandelion root because this stimulates the production of bile which carries toxins out of the liver. Don't buy dandelion coffee in a jar because it probably contains lactose, which is a form of sugar. Instead, buy a packet of dandelion root (obtainable either roasted or unroasted) and, if you have any coffee-making equipment, grind the root pieces and then make in the same way as 'proper' coffee, using a filter jug, percolator, etc. (Don't make like instant coffee by just adding boiling water.) Otherwise, simply place two heaped teaspoons of the root into a saucepan with about nine cups of water (weaker or stronger as preferred), bring to the boil and simmer for 15 minutes. Heat up a cupful whenever you feel like a hot drink; it is really very pleasant and it is extremely helpful for the liver.

- Take a herbal supplement containing silymarin, or milk thistle, known for generations for its liver-supportive properties.

- If these simple steps still leave you feeling in a toxic state, it would be well worth considering a hair mineral analysis to show levels of toxic elements that may have accumulated in your body, as well as checking on your absorption of nutritional minerals. A nutritionist would advise you on what to do once you had the results. Useful laboratories for this test are BioMed Ltd in the UK and Great Smokies in the USA *(see Appendix B)*.

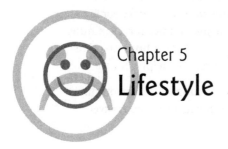

Chapter 5
Lifestyle

I realize, of course, that if your fatigue state is so severe that you are bed-bound, lifestyle hardly enters into consideration. However, reading this chapter might help you to make sense of at least part of the reason as to why you became ill in the first place, and it will also help you to be wise as your health begins to return.

There are in fact large numbers of people with diagnosed CFS who are somehow still managing to go to work or are struggling to take care of their families, and for those this chapter is essential reading.

When we are living our normal everyday lives, they often include some pretty negative habits which do us more harm than good. We have already talked about bad eating habits and how, for instance, tea and coffee actually block the absorption of many important minerals. Coffee drinkers, for example, are almost certain to be deficient in the mineral chromium because coffee carries it straight out of the body. There is probably not sufficient chromium in most people's diet to replace it, yet this mineral is essential for the regulation of the body's sugar stores. Without it, the control of sugar in the blood goes haywire so it is quite possible that hypoglycaemia and even late-onset diabetes might develop, slowly but surely, simply by drinking coffee! Not only this, but the stimulants in coffee and tea are addictive and set up a dependency on them which needs higher and higher levels of stimulation in order to avoid chronic headaches, exhaustion or feelings of jitteriness.

Other addictions, too, place an enormous strain on the body – alcohol, nicotine, the so-called 'recreational' drugs and also medical drugs like tranquillizers and sleeping pills. None of these do much to encourage the efficient working of our various body systems!

Then there is the question of rest and relaxation, both of which are essential for a healthy mind and body. If there is such a thing as a CFS 'type', it could well be a person with lots of 'drive', who overworks and is motivated by ambitions of achievement – hence the origin of the title 'Yuppie Flu'! To workaholics, sleep is just a necessary nuisance and relaxing with a book or watching television with the family is regarded as a sheer waste of time.

But the body is designed to need rest at regular intervals, and this is especially important when it has repairs to carry out. It is essential that when you are recovering from illness you should have early nights (late evening is *not* the time you should be watching TV!) in a comfortable bed. Even if insomnia is a problem, enjoy the fact that your body is warm and rested and that you can read a novel or listen to an audiotape. Aim to get up in the morning at a reasonable time, so that your lifestyle habits are as close to normal as you can make them. Lying in till noon only means that it will be harder to sleep at night. Of course, you should rest in the day-time as needed, but try to have a routine of meals at the same time as the others in your household. If you can eat with them, all well and good, but if you find it too tiring to talk and eat at the same time, sit quietly in a favourite chair and appreciate the food you're eating.

Relaxation is something you can develop. You can learn to appreciate listening to various types of music, or you can dabble with watercolour painting or pastel drawing or with embroidery or tapestry. I had one CFS client who had made some really wonderful tapestry wall-hangings, and her special Christmas cards were all hand-made in cross-stitch embroidery. It was good for her to be engrossed in this work, even though she could manage only a little at a time, and it was also good for her to be pleased with the end-results and to see the joy they brought to others. One hobby I would not recommend you take up is oil painting. The smell of white spirit which is used for thinning the paints and for cleaning brushes can be pretty noxious to many people!

Before you were ill, were you once a very active individual? Can you look back now and see how your body was abused through lack of adequate rest to help it cope with your demanding lifestyle? Did you ever make time for yourself to enjoy a relaxing hobby? Now is the opportunity to discover something which you would enjoy learning to do, so that you can keep it up and make time for it when you are once again well enough to live an active life.

Exercise can also be relaxing, especially in the fresh air, provided it is not undertaken with too much 'drive' or over-riding desire to achieve. Just exercise for the fun of it! Again, if you are too ill now, it is something to look forward to in the future. The body needs exercise for many reasons, not least because physical movement is the only way we have of mobilizing toxins around the lymphatic system so that they can be eliminated from the body via the bloodstream. Lack of exercise means that toxins are likely to stay in us for a lot longer than is helpful, giving rise to feelings of being 'out of sorts' even in a normally healthy person.

It is good to be determined to beat the illness, and every sufferer should continue to look forward to one day being well but, at the same time, it is important to *accept* the present situation while it lasts in order to have an inner peace. Frustration and impatience are added stresses, and these alone are sufficient to put a load on the immune system and slow down the healing process. We all need to learn to pace ourselves, even when we are well; when we are ill, rest and relaxation are essential to recovery.

ACTION PLAN

1   For each fatigue-sufferer, whether mobile or bed-bound, it is essential to take stock of your present diet and to eliminate junk foods and all addictive substances like tea, coffee, cola, chocolate and cocoa. If you think you don't actually need to follow the anti-candida diet in Chapter 17, turn to Chapter 20 to find guidelines for a good, general healthy eating plan. (Even if you are on an anti candida regime, this is what you will be aiming for eventually.)

2   Alcohol and nicotine both count as negative lifestyle factors!

3   If you are hooked on any type of drug, whether medical or recreational, talk to your doctor about help for breaking the addiction. There are in fact some excellent herbal supplements available to replace sleeping pills or tranquillizers (e.g. Valerian, Passiflora) but even so you will need your doctor's advice on how to wean yourself off the drugs.

4   If you are mobile and able to live a fairly normal life, take some time to consider your lifestyle. Ask yourself how much rest you are allowing yourself, including how many hours of sleep at night. How much time do you take to relax by yourself or to spend with your partner or family? Do you ever go to the cinema or theatre? Do you ever visit an art gallery? Do you have a hobby to help you unwind? If not, think about something you would like to take up and borrow a book from the library to tell you how to get started. Ask yourself, too, whether you get enough (or any!) exercise. Even though you

might find it a struggle to get through the day, it's quite possible that you would feel better for a 10-minute walk to work in the morning instead of taking the car or the bus. Another short walk at lunchtime would help you to unwind in the middle of your working day and would be far better for you than sitting around with your colleagues and possibly suffering the effects of passive smoking. You don't have to be ambitious about how much exercise you do, as long as you make a start, don't overstretch yourself – and enjoy it!

5   If exercise is out of the question because you are simply too ill, ask someone who cares for you to gently bend and straighten your arms and legs a few times each day. Even these small assisted movements will encourage toxins to circulate in your lymphatic system so that they can leave your body via your bloodstream. In addition, a build-up of lactic acid in the muscles is often responsible for making them ache, and gently stretching the muscles will help to offload this acid waste.

6   Also if you are too ill to take any form of exercise, make sure you have something to look forward to and enjoy – perhaps a story on an audiotape at a set time of day, following your afternoon nap, or a favourite weekly radio programme. Ask for a sketch pad and pencil, and see what you can manage to draw – if only for a few minutes while you are propped up in bed. Let there be some pleasure, an enthusiasm in your life, to replace the morbidity and frustration which otherwise take over with negative effects on your mind – and on your immune system. I remember times when I was at my lowest ebb, overwhelmed by sickness and anxiety, that my husband would sit with me and play game after game of Battleships with pencils and paper – a simple game that engrossed me for a while and helped to get me through the low point. It really did help!

7 When living through CFS, there are two sides to the coin which need to be held in balance. It is essential to hold on to faith for your future healing and well-being. Never lose sight of it. At the same time, on a daily basis it is essential that you fully accept your present circumstances just as they are in order to avoid suffering constant frustration and a lack of peace. Try to find ways of making the best of the situation while it lasts by building into your life some simple means of pleasure, enjoyment and even fulfilment.

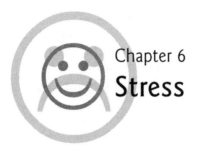

Chapter 6

Stress

What exactly is stress, and what does it do to us? Does it really have a part to play in chronic fatigue? Many fatigue sufferers don't take kindly to that idea; understandably, they resent the implied suggestion that they are mentally unwell, that their illness is 'all in the mind'. Many have been angered by the words, 'You'd be fine if you would just pull yourself together and get on with life'. It is frequently incredibly difficult to find someone to take their illness seriously. 'Reducing' their physical problems to a mental cause is therefore not the sort of help they welcome or think they need.

And yet . . . and yet. It is an undeniable fact that the body *is* affected by the mind. Consider how your knees knock or you have to rush to the lavatory when you are nervous, or your face goes red when you are embarrassed. If you have a shock, your face goes pale and your legs give way. If you are anxious, you tremble. These are very obvious links between the body and the mind but underlying them is the fact that any form of stress puts a load on the immune system by disrupting normal function of the adrenal hormones, and there are definite recorded changes in the immune response when a person is depressed or affected by a major life event, and at such times allergic reactions are much more likely to occur.

Both psychological and stressful social factors can have a strong influence on CFS. Psychological factors which count as stress can include emotional strain, anxiety or depression, time pressure, frustration, anger, perfectionism, being daunted by an overwhelming work-load and feeling out of control or unfulfilled. Social factors might include any major event which has brought shock or distress such as bereavement, redundancy, trauma or accident. They also include everyday things like shift work, pollution and extremes of environmental temperature (like stepping out of an over-heated building into an icy cold wind). Some people, of course, have a greater ability to cope than others, and research suggests that people who cope badly experience greater immune changes when confronted with a shock than do those who cope well, so that individual personality and psychology can play a part in suppressing immunity which is as significant as stress itself. This is partly due to previous experience, the 'programming' which has taken place in our minds as a response to life's events.

Our ability to cope emotionally also depends on how we are feeling physically. Stress is not actually what goes on 'out there' in our lives; it is our inward reaction to those situations and circumstances. For instance, if you were to discover a splinter in a finger but otherwise felt quite well, you would simply squeeze it out and forget about it. But if you were ill in bed with a bad bout of flu, the splinter could easily become a source of major anxiety; 'If I can't get it out, I'll die of septicaemia!' You might remain obsessed with it for hours, making the poor finger more and more sore by squeezing it and prodding it with a needle. A vicious circle then sets in because a stressful reaction leads to a weakened immune system, and a weakened immune system leads to more sickness and a greater inability to cope, which in turn leads to more anxiety and depression which further weaken the immune system, making it less and less able to fight off disease or allergy.

In their book *Nutritional Medicine*, Drs Stephen Davies and Alan Stewart state that people undergoing stress are more likely to develop food intolerances and also that allergies are more pronounced when patients are anxious or stressed but less of a problem when they are relaxed. It is impossible to deny the very strong links which exist between the body and the mind so it is important that everything possible should be done to sort out situations causing worry or depression and, more than that, to overcome negative attitudes towards those situations.

We all need some stimulation or we decline into apathy, but each of us has an optimum stress level beyond which the stimulation does more harm than good. Stress can be anger, fear, excitement or frustration, any of which will have a stimulant effect upon the adrenal glands – as do certain foods and drinks such as sugar, salt, alcohol, tea, coffee, chocolate, cocoa and cola drinks, and also cigarettes.

Whether or not stresses and strains were part of the picture before the onset of chronic fatigue, there is no doubt that the illness brings its own overwhelming stresses. This needs to be acknowledged and ways must be found to alleviate the situation as far as possible in order to reduce the stress load on the immune system. Unfortunately, since excitement over-stimulates the adrenals just as much as anxiety, you might feel just as ill after watching a good football match on television as if you had spent the time worrying about the bills that still need paying. It might make for a dull life for the moment, but it is better to keep your emotions on an even keel than get worked up about anything at all.

Of course, if we accept the fact that immune function can be depressed by negative psychological and emotional factors, then we need to agree that the opposite must also be true – that our immune systems can be helped to work more efficiently if we are happy and can develop an inner peace and serenity of outlook. I have known several people (including me!) who turned a definite corner towards recovery once they found they could off-load their fears and anxieties on God, and in their place received faith for the future.

One effect of stress is that it triggers the release of adrenalin which in turn organizes the release of the body's sugar stores from the liver into the blood, and this has several knock-on effects relating to other pieces of cargo on our immune ship, so stress reactions need to be reduced as much as possible. This initial release of adrenalin is known as the 'alarm response'. It registers the alarm which would have been felt by our cave-man ancestor when he walked round a rock and found himself in the path of a great big woolly mammoth. The shock would have led to an immediate release of adrenalin by his adrenal hormones, and this in turn would have stimulated the release of his body's sugar stores into his bloodstream. A surge of blood-sugar gives rise to a burst of energy, so great-great-great-great-grandpa would then have had strength either to stand up and fight the beast or turn around and run away as fast as his legs could carry him! We, of course, when confronted with an infuriatingly slow red traffic light, simply drum our fingers on the steering wheel – which burns up very little of the excess sugar poured into our blood as a result of frustration, so it stays in our bodies doing harm! (This is why exercise, where possible, is an important first-aid treatment for stressful feelings – a brisk walk or exercise session works wonders at burning up the excess sugar, but this is cold comfort to someone who struggles just to sit up in bed each day. However, simple relaxation techniques also help body systems to get back to normal. Tense your muscles as hard as you can and then relax, starting with your feet and ending with your face. Or just clench your fists and then relax.)

This sugar-surge only happens when sudden stress or a shock triggers the release of adrenalin. So what happens to the adrenals when stress has been long-term and unremitting – as sadly is too often the case in this day and age of marriage break-ups, job redundancies, housing problems, teenage children going off the rails, and so on?

In this situation, the adrenal glands becoming increasingly over-worked and then exhausted. They obviously need more help, which the body very cleverly provides. When adrenalin is no longer man enough for the job, the adrenals release two other types of stress hormone called cortisol and DHEA (dehydroepiandrosterone). In a healthy situation, cortisol is released in a regular daily cycle (known as the Circadian rhythm), which starts at a high point first thing in the morning and ends the day by being low. This is necessary if we are to experience fully-restorative sleep at night. However, if stress continues after the alarm response, more and more stimulation is needed to keep the adrenals working, so there may be cravings for harmful stimulants like sugar, tea, coffee, alcohol and cigarettes. The adrenal glands stimulate the release of more cortisol while producing less DHEA and, if the situation is prolonged, the body's resources are used for making even more cortisol instead of producing DHEA, which then drops lower and lower. At the same time, the pituitary and hypothalamus glands in the brain become less sensitive and remain unaware of the high level of cortisol being produced, so they continue to send messages to the adrenal glands to release even more of it.

Eventually, however, as the adrenal glands become increasingly worn down by all the effort they are having to make, they start to produce less cortisol and at the same time levels of DHEA start to rise. When this occurs, the adrenals are well on the way to being truly exhausted and, if stressful situations continue unremittingly, one day the adrenals will have extreme difficulty in producing even small amounts of either cortisol or DHEA. In that situation, the body is unable to cope with the smallest amount of stress, and chronic ill-health is unavoidable.

Even in the initial stages, irregularities in output of the adrenal hormones can have many knock-on effects, exerting an unhealthy influence on metabolism and energy production, muscle and joint function, the strength of bones and of the immune system, the quality of sleep and the health of the skin and its ability to regenerate. Quite often, hypothyroid symptoms such as fatigue, low body temperature and others which you can read about in Chapter 8 – 'Inefficient Thyroid Function', are actually due to adrenal fatigue. One frequently-experienced symptom is a sense of 'driven-ness'. It becomes impossible to rest and you have to keep active and stimulated all the time. If you go to the cinema, you choose an edge-of-the-seat thriller rather than a relaxed romantic comedy, or if you go on holiday you choose to water-ski or shoot the rapids rather than lie back by the sea with a sunshade and a slow-paced historical novel. You've gone way past the point of being able to unwind – but unless you do, your driven-ness will one day become adrenal exhaustion.

The problem is that this situation does not go away even if your stressful circumstances are one day happily resolved. The over-stretched adrenals cannot suddenly ping back like a piece of elastic; they continue to produce levels of cortisol and DHEA which are either too high or too low and your mind still constantly urges your body to keep doing more than it should – until you find that you are no longer able to sleep properly or wake refreshed, that you are always catching colds or flu, that your joints and muscles ache most of the time, that you are depressed, that you have developed skin problems, that your temperature control has gone haywire, and so on. The situation becomes a vicious circle because ill-health in itself is stressful, and inflammation of any type also places a load on the adrenal stress hormones.

It can be helpful in this situation to undertake a diagnostic test using saliva specimens collected at set times during the day, which show the levels and behaviour of cortisol and DHEA compared with a normal reference range. This pattern will not vary depending on stressful circumstances on any given day because it shows the long-term behaviour of the two hormones, a pattern that will have developed over a period of time and is unaffected by the daily output of adrenalin when it is released to cope with additional short-term stress. The laboratory I have used for some years is Diagnos-Tech, which is based in the USA, but easily accessible by practitioners in the UK through an address in Wales *(see Appendix B)*.

The laboratory report comes back with a couple of graphs, one showing the daily output of cortisol as plotted against a fairly wide reference range of 'normal' cortisol production, and the other showing the daytime output of cortisol in relation to the output of DHEA, which also is shown against its own reference range. If DHEA is low, this may in itself indicate adrenal depletion but it is actually the relationship between the levels of the two hormones which is more significant. You can tell from these figures whether stress is still causing an increase in cortisol, in which case the adrenals are still capable of adapting to cope with stress to some extent, or whether it has already led to a state of adrenal dysfunction that is causing both the hormones to fall to levels which are inadequate for their task.

With all this information, it becomes possible to regulate both cortisol and DHEA in whichever ways are necessary, not only by taking appropriate nutritional supplements but by knowing at which times of day they are needed in order to manipulate the irregular daily cycle back to a normal reference range. For instance, small amounts of liquorice taken at the right time of day can help to increase the output of cortisol. This needs to be taken with some care and preferably with professional guidance, because liquorice can have the effect of increasing blood pressure. (This can be avoided by also supplementing potassium.) On the other hand, cortisol which is too high can be reduced by taking a food supplement containing phosphatidyl serine at appropriate times of day. This is an expensive product but it has been shown that taking a supplement providing nutrients which are precursors to phosphatidyl serine can be just as effective, and this is a cheaper way of achieving the same objective. When overall cortisol output is very high indeed, this situation can be tackled by taking the amino acid L-Tyrosine in addition to phosphatidyl serine precursors.

People in the UK who are suffering from low DHEA have more of a problem than their American cousins because DHEA is available in Britain only on prescription by a medical practitioner, and not many doctors seem to have experience of it. In America, it is still available as an over-the-counter product. However, Siberian ginseng, which is known as an adaptogen because it helps the adrenals to adapt, has shown itself to be almost, if not equally, as effective as taking DHEA itself. Most of my UK clients show a slow but steady increase in their output of DHEA if they have been taking Siberian ginseng for a while, and later have a follow-up diagnostic test to see what has been achieved.

A common effect of high cortisol is that it impedes the body's production of the secretory antibodies which line the intestinal wall, known as SIgA. These particular antibodies may actually be called the first line of defence of the immune system because if SIgA is low, this opens the way for the bloodstream to be invaded by bacteria, viruses, fungi, parasites, allergens and toxins from the gastrointestinal tract. It is therefore very useful that the same diagnostic saliva test can actually show the levels of SIgA present in the saliva specimen and that this reflects the levels on the intestinal lining, which gives a fair idea of how effectively the immune system is able to hold back potential invaders as they try to make their way through the gut wall. Apart from reducing stressful factors and taking steps to reduce cortisol or regulate the adrenal hormones in other ways, it can be helpful to take supplements which encourage the production of intestinal mucus, thus encouraging the secretory antibodies to spread. A specially treated form of liquorice that has been deglycyrrhinized is useful in this respect and, unlike the untreated liquorice used for stimulating cortisol production, it does not have the potential problem of causing an increase in blood pressure. Cabagin (also known as vitamin U) from cabbage is another substance which helps to soothe the intestinal lining and enhance the growth and effectiveness of natural lactic bacteria in the gut – all necessary for the adequate production of secretory intestinal antibodies.

When under stress, it is obvious that the adrenal glands need to be supported nutritionally so taking a few simple supplements can be extremely helpful. In particular, vitamins C and B_5 should be taken, together with a B Complex to replace all the other B vitamins which are being burned up. In the early stages of stress before adrenal function has been stretched too far, this nutritional support is possibly the only supplementation you need to consider for supporting your adrenals. You might also like to try taking herbal supplements of St John's Wort or Valerian to help over-ride depression and anxiety and keep your moods on an even keel.

You can do a surprising amount to support your adrenal glands and therefore strengthen your immune system by taking notice of the levels of protein and carbohydrate which you eat at every single meal and every single snack. The ideal ratio of carbohydrate to protein should be approximately 2:1, measured in grams, calories or simply by size. A rough guide is to measure enough food to cover the palm of your hand; a palm-sized portion of protein to two palm-sized portions of carbohydrate. You probably know that when a nutritionist talks about carbohydrate, we don't mean refined carbohydrates like white flour and sugar, but complex carbohydrates like whole grains, vegetables and fruit. However, you should avoid all fruit if you happen to be on the anti-candida diet *(Chapter 17)* and in any case don't have fruit on its own because it is mainly carbohydrate, which means that you immediately lose the balance with protein that you are aiming for. You can achieve this 2:1 ratio quite easily by having for instance one portion of fish (protein) with two portions of vegetables (carbohydrate), or one portion of black-eye beans (beans and pulses provide excellent protein when combined with a whole grain) with whole-grain rice and a vegetable (carbohydrates), or egg or cottage cheese (protein) with a wheat or rye cracker and a tomato (both carbohydrate). This way of eating also helps to control blood sugar levels and even improves metabolism, so that it becomes easier to lose weight if you need to, or to increase your energy output. For further reading on the interesting effects of this way of balancing your food, see *The Zone* by Dr Barry Sears.

Adrenal function can also be helped by appropriate exercise. Depending on how active you are able to be, this is certainly worth bearing in mind, especially if you can go for walks. However, if as yet you are too ill to be able to contemplate exercise, don't worry – it will be possible all in good time! This advice also needs to be weighed against the fact that exercise stirs up toxins in the lymphatic system so that they are tipped rather too hurriedly into the bloodstream, where they can give rise to many unpleasant symptoms. In someone who is following an anti-candida programme, for instance, it can lead to an increase in die-off reaction *(see Chapter 12 – 'Die-off'!)*. Exercise therefore needs to be monitored carefully, depending on the current situation.

It might take a few months to nudge the adrenal stress hormones back into line, but the effort is well worthwhile in terms of increased immune function, let alone the benefits experienced in reduced depression, insomnia and all the other problems which occur when adrenal hormones are out of balance. I strongly suggest that, if you have a suspicion (or even a certainty) that stressful circumstances in the present or the past, however long ago, have left you with battered and dysfunctional adrenal glands, it would be well worth your while to seek out a nutritionist who could arrange an Adrenal Stress Index diagnostic test for you and then prepare a tailor-made programme to help restore your adrenals to a state of health in which they can help your body to cope with stress efficiently and easily.

And of course it must still be remembered that, even though a diagnostic test to show the levels and behaviour of adrenal stress hormones is extremely helpful, it is also essential to take steps to sort out your lifestyle and existing problems in practical terms as far as you possibly can, in order to minimize the effects of on-going stress. There are many ways in which a nutritionist can give advice to help with recovery from physical and even mental or emotional illness, but some of life's problems will never be solved by nutritional therapy alone. However, a trusting and supportive relationship with a caring practitioner can still go a long way towards lightening the stress load on the immune system. In addition, a carefully-calculated supplement programme which has been tailor-made for a specific individual can do a great deal to improve their stress reactions, which means that they will also find an increased ability to cope.

The following Action Plan for minimizing the effects of stress should be helpful to you.

ACTION PLAN

Some nutritional tips:

1 **Cut right down on animal fat, but eat plenty of oily fish, nuts and seeds**. Try a delicious salad dressing every day made of a good unrefined oil such as sunflower, linseed or safflower, mixed with a little fresh lemon juice.

2 **Take Calcium pantothenate (vitamin B$_5$) to give your adrenal glands some nutritional support.** It needs to be taken with the other B vitamins so look for a good multivitamin supplement that contains these and other nutrients at useful levels. (Make sure the label says that the

product contains no yeast, lactose or other forms of sugar.) Take a minimum of 50 mg of B$_5$, but you can safely take it up to 300 mg or even more, with practitioner guidance.)

3 **Take good levels of vitamin C.** How much is a 'good level'? It varies from person to person, and for each person it varies from day to day! A minimum of 1000 mg (1 gram) would be helpful to your adrenals, but probably 3000 mg (3 grams) would be even better. It all depends on how much it takes to reach 'bowel tolerance', in other words the level which causes a loose motion. Many people have a temporary requirement of extremely high levels, and bowel tolerance is the only guideline there is as to when you have had enough. A word of caution; it is better not to take more than 1 gram of vitamin C if you are taking the contraceptive pill or any form of hormone therapy, as it might increase the risk of potential adverse effects from the hormone treatment. And always take vitamin C as part of a good multivitamin/mineral programme *(see Chapter 3 – 'Nutritional Deficiencies').*

4 **Take 1000 mg (1 gram) Siberian ginseng daily** if you are suffering from long-term stress, as it helps the adrenals to adapt. Take it with breakfast and have regular breaks. I suggest two months on and two weeks off.

5 **Try taking a herbal supplement containing St John's Wort** to help reduce depression and keep your emotions on an even keel. (Don't take it if you are on Prozac or other MAOI antidepressants, or Seroxat or other SSRI antidepressants.)

Some practical tips for long-term stress control:

1 Limit your working time to 10 hours per day, five days per week at most.

2   Keep at least one-and-a-half days a week completely free of routine work.

3   Make sure you use this free time to cultivate a relaxing hobby, do something creative or take exercise, preferably in the fresh air.

4   Try to adopt a relaxed manner. For instance, walk and talk more slowly. A useful idea is to act as if you *were* a relaxed person, like a game.

5   Avoid obvious pressures, such as taking on too many commitments.

6   Learn to see when a problem is somebody else's responsibility, and don't try to carry it all by yourself.

7   If you have an emotional problem – or even a practical one – which you cannot solve alone, seek advice.

8   Concentrate on one task at a time, and focus all your attention on the present.

9   Learn to say what is on your mind instead of suppressing it. You don't have to be aggressive – just state your point of view clearly.

10   If someone says something nice to you, or about you, be grateful and believe it!

11   Don't be too proud to receive help or sympathy when it is offered and you need it.

12   Think about all the stresses in your life and make a list of them. Set out to find a positive attitude to things which cannot be changed but, if change *is* possible, take action! Don't let things wear you down.

13   If you have faith, use it. If your faith has lapsed, revive it. If you have no faith, consider the difference it would make to your life to know that prayers can be answered!

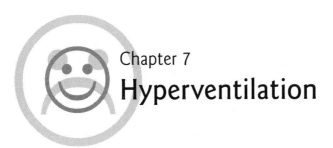

Chapter 7

Hyperventilation

I include the subject of hyperventilation immediately after the chapter on stress because people very often hyperventilate when they are feeling anxious. This particular piece of cargo has rather found its way into this book through the back door, so to speak, because it has even less to do with a nutritional approach to overcoming CFS than the chapter on Lifestyle, which did at least make some comments about negative dietary factors! However, I believe it would not be right to leave it out of any discussion about the fatigue syndrome because it is almost certainly responsible for being a larger piece of cargo than most of us realize.

What is hyperventilation? It means simply 'overbreathing' or breathing in a way which is too fast and too deep. Breathing like this quickly lowers the level of carbon dioxide in the blood which alters the body's acid/alkali balance which in turn affects the way our nerves fire and interact with one another. It can lead to muscle ache and fatigue, giddiness, faintness, numbness, loss of consciousness, blurred vision, headaches, nausea, weak limbs, inability to walk, trembling, palpitations, chest pain, fatigue and panic attacks. You can see how this set of symptoms, if experienced continuously, could quite easily be mistaken for CFS, irrespective of what else might be going on in the body.

Unfortunately, quite often a vicious circle is established. Let's say you once had a panic attack in a certain place, perhaps in a shopping precinct. After that, your mind associates that unpleasant experience with the place you were in at the time, so next time you go there it isn't surprising that you start feeling anxious as you recall what happened before – and because you are anxious, your breathing quickens and you also probably take a few deep breaths as you fight to stay calm. In other words, you hyperventilate. Unfortunately, overbreathing in this way will automatically trigger both the physical and mental symptoms that you were so anxious to avoid – including panic! As soon as you recognize what is happening, you need to find somewhere to sit and make yourself breathe quietly, concentrating particularly on slow but shallow breaths. If you are in a suitable place where you won't feel too conspicuous, it is helpful to breathe into your cupped hands or into a paper bag for a few moments. In this way you re-inhale the carbon dioxide which you just breathed out, and this reverses the symptoms and defuses the panic attack.

Hyperventilation is not always associated with stress; it may simply be due to bad habits or to long-standing tension due to illness, so again there can be a vicious circle. It is important for fatigue sufferers to learn how to breathe slowly and shallowly and to relax their muscles. Often when we are ill we sit huddled up with our arms folded and our shoulders stooped and clenched. In that position, our breathing may not be deep but it will certainly be too fast. It is therefore not surprising that symptoms of hyperventilation, so similar to many which we associate with CFS, continue to be experienced. We need to learn new breathing habits, and this takes time and practice. Frequent or chronic hyperventilation increases stress levels and has the very opposite effect from the inner calm and serenity which it is so important to cultivate when the body is in need of healing.

We have probably all been taught at some time in our lives that it is important for us to breathe deeply, to fill our lungs with good fresh air so that we take in plenty of oxygen, and to empty our lungs of carbon dioxide so that we breathe out all the waste products. Surprisingly, it now appears that we have all been badly taught! Two books have been written, each of them explaining the discoveries and work of a Russian professor, Konstantin Buteyko. The first one I came across was *Freedom from Asthma* by Alexander Stalmatski, and a year or so later I found *Breathing Free* by Teresa Hale. They each explain the problems caused by over-breathing and, although there are some differences in their corrective approach to it, both techniques are geared towards learning a new way of breathing which will mean that the body takes in less oxygen and retains more carbon dioxide. That does not seem to make sense, does it? Yet Professor Buteyko's work with literally millions of cases proves that it does make sense and that, simply by learning new ways of breathing, not only can asthma be dramatically improved but many other types of health problem can be remarkably overcome.

I attended a weekend of training by Alexander Stalmatski in London. My reason for going was two-fold: to accompany my friend Janet who is a long-term asthma sufferer, heavily dependent on steroid medication for it, and to see for myself what this was about. At the end of the weekend, after five sessions of training, Janet was able to run up the steps at our local railway station and telephone her husband to collect us – without even panting, let alone gasping for breath! What is more, this lady who had taken medication for asthma for something like 22 years had not once had to use her bronchodilator inhaler over the entire weekend. I was definitely impressed – and I am not one who is easily persuaded to take strange new ideas on board, believe me!

Teresa Hale introduces her book by explaining what is wrong with our understanding that it is good to breathe deeply in order to increase our oxygen intake and off-load carbon dioxide. In fact, she says, the reverse is true because the more we breathe (whether deeply or quickly), the less oxygen actually reaches the cells of our body because, however much oxygen might be available, our bodies cannot use it unless there is also a certain amount of carbon dioxide around. She therefore describes healthy breathing as being quiet and shallow, so that our chests barely move.

If learning to breathe properly can improve asthma in just a couple of days, what can it do for other health problems? Professor Buteyko discovered that hyperventilation lies at the root of nearly 200 other disorders – including CFS. This is not too surprising when you consider the various effects of having too little carbon dioxide. In terms of muscle aches alone, Teresa Hale explains:

> Without balanced breathing, oxygen in the cell is not released into the muscle, causing the muscle tiredness of chronic fatigue. With balanced breathing, the oxygen in the cell is released into the muscle.

She also explains that hyperventilation can prevent blood flow to the brain, leading to dizziness and loss of concentration and memory. Other signs include weakness, exhaustion, sleep disturbance, breathlessness, heartburn, cramps and pins and needles. Do you recognize some of these?

In making Professor Buteyko's research and findings accessible to us, I believe that Alexander Stalmatski and Teresa Hale have opened the door to improvements in health at very many levels – and not just for asthma sufferers. I have realized for a long time that hyperventilation justified being recognized as a piece of cargo that is frequently found on a weakened *Immunity* ship, and these two writers have confirmed my thinking and sharpened up the picture of what actually occurs when we over-breathe – and shown to what a large extent most of us are guilty of doing it.

There is no doubt that hyperventilation leads to an increase of the symptoms of CFS, and then chronic fatigue makes our breathing worse and so we are caught in a vicious circle. But we ourselves have the key to the lock!

Learning to break and replace a lifetime's unhealthy breathing habits and learning to do it properly could possibly give you just the lift you're needing while the nutritional steps you're about to take get on with the work of off-loading other pieces of cargo which have encouraged your immune ship to flounder. Start to throw off this one piece of cargo – the one in the extra-long box with its name written all down one side – right now!

ACTION PLAN

- Of the two books mentioned, I strongly recommend that you acquire a copy of *Breathing Free* by Teresa Hale. It is in clear print, easy to read and understand, and most interesting! Various breathing techniques are simply explained, with helpful diagrams, for use in different situations. For instance, there's a technique for dealing with panic attacks and a calming technique for reducing daily stress levels. There is even a daily self-care programme for healthy people and a technique to use when you have a cold, flu or hayfever.

Such a small amount of effort is required – it *has* to be worth trying! As my friend Janet remarked, 'All this plus optimum nutrition – who could go wrong?' However, Janet also makes the point that she has no doubt of the part played in asthma by an overgrowth of the common yeast, *Candida albicans (see Chapter 10 – 'Gut Dysbiosis')* because of the improvement she has experienced by following the anti-candida four-point plan *(see Chapter 11)* – yet no mention is made of this in either of the books on breathing techniques. It's worth bearing in mind again that no one approach is likely to have the whole answer. Even if you do hyperventilate, it is almost certainly just one of the possible pieces of cargo on your *Immunity* ship.

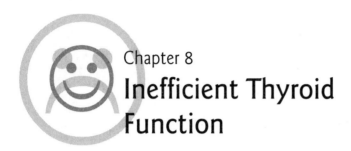

Chapter 8

Inefficient Thyroid Function

The thyroid is the largest gland in the body. It affects every major organ and stimulates the repair of all our body's cells and the manufacture of its enzymes. It has a major influence on hormonal function so that, apart from anything else, an under-active thyroid can lead to problems of menstrual irregularities. Diagnos-Techs, one of America's leading diagnostic laboratories, states that the second most commonly diagnosed endocrine disorders are those of the thyroid gland. (The first is diabetes.)

Every drop of our 10 pints or so of blood circulates through the thyroid gland every single hour, bringing with it the substances that the thyroid needs to do its work. If you don't produce enough thyroid hormones, everything in your body slows down – heartbeat, circulation, blood pressure, energy levels, metabolism and temperature. If you make too many thyroid hormones, everything in your body speeds up – like an old Charlie Chaplin film when it's run at the wrong speed! Your heartbeat and blood pressure increase, you overheat and produce lots of perspiration, and every system in your body is overactive.

The following lists show some of the major signs of thyroid imbalance:

Hypothyroid (underactive thyroid)

Fatigue and/or lethargy
Dry skin and/or hair
Intolerance to cold
Constipation
Facial swelling
Weight gain (though sometimes weight loss)
Painful periods
Other menstrual irregularities

Hyperthyroid (overactive thyroid)

Nervousness and/or anxiety
Palpitations and/or irregular heartbeat
Fatigue
Insomnia
Weight loss
Increased appetite
Diarrhoea
Increased sweating

You will see that fatigue occurs whether your thyroid is working too fast or too slowly. As a nutritionist, I am mostly concerned with looking for signs of an underactive or inefficient thyroid gland. This is because in my training I was taught that an overactive thyroid is often indicative of problems which need medical attention and are therefore outside the scope of nutritional intervention. However, Dr Stephen Langer in his book *Solved: the Riddle of Illness*, talks about his sense of horror when he recalls that, for the first half of the 20th century, it was standard surgical procedure to remove a thyroid gland, whether it was overproductive or under-productive, yet it is possible in many instances to correct unbalanced thyroid hormone production –

either too much or too little – merely by compensating for certain vitamin deficiencies. He argues that in many cases this is still all that needs to be done, and can actually be more effective than the pharmaceutical drugs which are commonly prescribed.

If your doctor orders a blood test to check out your thyroid function, the laboratory technician will be looking for the number of circulating thyroid hormones in the blood sample. However, if you feel cold most of the time, this is a clue that although there might be an adequate number of thyroid hormones swimming around in your blood, they are not actually working very efficiently.

This standard of thyroid efficiency may be tested by taking your underarm temperature first thing in the morning before you get out of bed, a procedure which is based on the work of Dr Broda Barnes and which forms the major content of Dr Langer's book. Your early-morning, under-arm temperature taken for two days will give a fair indication of what is happening, but of course doing it for a longer period of time would give a more realistic picture. The lowest end of 'normal' is 97.8°F or 36.5°C. See the following *Action Plan* for guidance on how to interpret your findings and what to do if the situation needs help.

Normally, with appropriate nutritional measures, a slow but steady rise in temperature readings will occur over a few months, indicating an improvement in thyroid efficiency and, almost certainly, at the same time there will be a decrease in many symptoms, including chilliness.

In many cases, low body temperature will not necessarily indicate a condition that would be medically diagnosed as an actual underactive thyroid. We are considering the possibility of what might be called a subclinical condition of thyroid inefficiency – which in itself, according to Dr Langer, can be responsible for chronic fatigue, aching in joints and muscles, depression, certain types of anaemia, recurrent infections and an inability to lose weight, showing that many symptoms of an underactive or even just a subclinically inefficient thyroid can be exactly the same as many of those which we associate with CFS.

An inefficient thyroid gland makes it extremely difficult to distinguish between the symptoms it is causing and those which might be due to other factors in the CFS ragbag. Obviously, nutritional steps should be taken to improve the situation if this is indicated by low body temperature, so that at least some of the symptoms in the overall condition may be eliminated or at least improved.

Dr Langer's approach to improving the situation is to prescribe desiccated thyroid preparation, but this type of glandular supplementation which is derived from animal glands is not the preferred way of working for many nutritionists. I have frequently found that a low body temperature will slowly but surely increase on a programme which includes a tailor-made food supplement programme, with some additional seaweed products providing iodine from either dulse or kelp.

ACTION PLAN

1 Read the following extract from *Solved: The Riddle of Illness*, by Dr Stephen Langer, and then do the temperature test as described:

'Your thyroid function needs checking.'

Their reactions could be summed up in the words: 'Not *another* test!' All of them had gone through exhaustive tests, including one for thyroid function, at a cost of hundreds of dollars.

'This won't cost you a cent,' I assured them. 'You can do the Barnes Basal Temperature Test yourself at home.'

They were puzzled. Who had ever heard of a no-cost test? Then I explained how to do it.

'Before going to bed tonight, shake down a thermometer.

Leave it on the bedside table. As soon as you wake up in the morning after a good night's sleep – no later – tuck the thermometer snugly in your armpit for ten minutes as you lie there.

'If your thyroid function is normal, your temperature should be in the range of 97.8 to 98.2 degrees Fahrenheit (36.5 to 36.7 degrees Centigrade). If it's lower, you are probably hypothyroid – your thyroid gland is underfunctioning – and your physical problems and related ones have probably been caused or at least influenced by that. The test should be done on two consecutive days.'

To the women I said, 'You can get the most accurate readings when you're menstruating, on the second and third day after your period starts.'

Reported results confirmed my suspicions: all were indeed hypothyroid.

So now you know how to do the Barnes Basal Temperature Test! Here's some more detail on how to interpret your findings, and also what you can do about them:

2 Take your early-morning, under-arm temperature on two consecutive days. If either of your temperature readings is below 97.8°F (36.5°C), take it again over a longer period of time, say a week, to see if it is low on a fairly regular basis. If it is not below 97.0°F (36.1°C), you will probably see improvements simply by taking a tailor-made supplement programme that includes your optimal levels of the B vitamins *(see Chapter 3 – 'Nutritional Deficiencies')*. There are some delicious seaweed products available in health-food stores, which would help to supply your body with thyroid-regulating iodine.

3 If your temperature readings are significantly below 97.8°F (36.5°C), you would definitely benefit by taking some iodine-providing supplements of kelp or dulse, and possibly also the

amino acid L-Tyrosine, but this should be taken under practitioner guidance.

4 If you take steps to improve your thyroid efficiency, take your early-morning temperature again for a couple of mornings every month or so. As it starts to increase, you will hopefully find that some of your symptoms also start to improve.

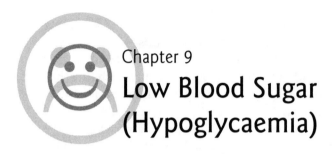

Chapter 9

Low Blood Sugar (Hypoglycaemia)

As with most of the other pieces of cargo on the immune ship that we have looked at so far, the symptoms of low blood sugar are virtually the same as those which you associate with CFS – dizziness, exhaustion, headache, weakness, fatigue, depression, anxiety, panic, energy slumps and so on. This means that if you have CFS but, unknown to you, low blood sugar (hypoglycaemia) has been one of your problems, improving your blood sugar balance will mean that at least some of your symptoms will actually feel quite a lot better, symptoms which you had previously thought of as just being part of CFS.

'I have CFS so of course I have energy slumps, headaches, dizziness, etc.', yet hypoglycaemia could have been responsible for any of those symptoms, at the same time weakening your immune system. Even if it is not the whole answer because other pieces of cargo are also weighing down the ship, correcting hypoglycaemia will prevent your blood sugar control from going down the slippery slope to diabetes – for that is what can happen.

I like to tell my clients to imagine a graph that indicates levels of sugar (glucose) in the blood. If you have a chronic condition of low blood sugar, every time you take in some sugar, the line on the graph will shoot up to a high point, indicating that you now have a very high level of sugar in your blood. This sugar-load happens whenever you eat something sweetened with sugar or something which quickly converts to glucose when you eat it (e.g. white flour, white rice) or whenever you stimulate your adrenal glands with tea, coffee, alcohol, cola drinks, chocolate or cigarettes. It also happens when your adrenals are stimulated by stress or excitement.

If your blood-sugar level stayed up at the high point on the graph, you would have a chronic condition of high blood sugar, which makes it a fairly safe bet that you are heading for diabetes. In order to avoid this happening, the body does something very clever. A message is sent to the pancreas telling it to release some insulin. Insulin helps the situation by encouraging sugar in the blood to be taken up sideways, so to speak, into the cells of the body. This means that the level of sugar left in the blood falls very low indeed, so the line on the graph plummets right down to a low point. When sugar levels are really low, you experience some particularly unpleasant symptoms. You might feel dizzy and faint, or have a headache, feel irritable or depressed, have a panic attack, become aggressive or just feel plain exhausted.

So, as with an addiction when we talked about allergies in Chapter 2, you reach for something to give you a 'lift', something which you have found from experience will pick you up quite quickly. It might be tea or coffee, a biscuit, some chocolate, a doughnut or a glass of beer or sherry! Quite soon the symptoms pass, you feel better and able to cope again – but the new-found energy doesn't last. Why? Because your raised blood sugar has triggered a message to be sent to your pancreas once more to stimulate the release of yet more insulin, so once again the line on the graph has plummeted down to a low point. And what do you do then? Have another cup of coffee or another bar of chocolate! You can perhaps see from this simple explanation that your need for sugar or stimulants will actually increase the more you continue to trigger the release of insulin.

When we talk about blood sugar, we are talking about energy. The picture of peaks and troughs of blood sugar shown on the graph reflects the yo-yo effect in your energy levels throughout the day. I can't tell you how many of my clients have nodded their heads in agreement as they have recognized themselves in my description of out-of-control blood sugar levels! As the situation continues, the poor old pancreas over-reacts and becomes trigger-happy in its release of insulin, so the line on the graph cavorts across the page, jumping from mountain peak to valley trough and back again, on and on and on. The parts of the body which are trying to control the situation become increasingly exhausted and the situation grows steadily worse. Eventually, the pancreas itself becomes so worn out that it is unable to produce more insulin, so there is nothing to help the sugar level fall, and that is the point when late-onset diabetes sets in. Yet it could have been totally avoided. How?

If you change your diet and eat only those foods which either release no sugar at all or else release it only slowly, you can change the line on your graph from peaks and troughs to a gentle, undulating curve of slight ups and downs. You need to avoid table sugar (sucrose) entirely, so that means all foods containing sugar (sweets, cakes, biscuits, sweetened cereals – in fact most packaged goods including savoury ones, because even these will usually contain some sugar!). Even natural sugar like honey should be avoided for the time being, and fruit should be kept to an absolute minimum because of its own natural sugar content (fructose) – in fact, you are best without it for now. You must certainly avoid all types of fruit juice (even pure ones) for this same reason and, if you ever do want to go back to it, always make sure it is well-diluted with water. Incidentally, artificial sweeteners must also be avoided, as should all refined grains (white flour, white rice, cornflour) because they quickly digest into glucose. All stimulants must also be avoided because of their effect on the adrenal glands which triggers the release of the body's sugar stores back into your blood – so that means no tea, coffee, cola, chocolate or alcohol. Even salt is a stimulant and should be drastically reduced.

It helps to eat at frequent intervals so that you 'catch' the line on the graph before it drops too low. Besides having regular meals, plan to have the right sort of snack mid-morning and mid-afternoon, and always have something at bedtime because blood sugar levels hit their lowest point in the small hours of the night. It is not uncommon for low blood sugar to mimic a heart attack at 3 am. And never, ever, go without breakfast because once you start to expend some energy, your sugar levels for the rest of the day will never be able to catch up.

Apart from making some changes and adjustments to your diet, you also need to take specific vitamin and mineral supplements. An important substance called Glucose Tolerance Factor (GTF) is made by the liver and is essential for controlling blood sugar levels. It is heavily dependent on receiving good levels of chromium and vitamin B_3, so these two nutrients should appear in your supplement programme. Other important vitamins and minerals are vitamins B_5, B_6 and C, and zinc and manganese. These minerals also help to support the adrenal glands, which will have been weakened by erratic blood sugar control, and weak adrenals mean weak immunity, so apart from removing or alleviating some symptoms by dealing with low blood sugar, it will actually help your immune system in its overall fight to throw off CFS. And the pancreas, once it no longer needs to pump out insulin all day every day, will be able to take a deep breath and say, 'Ah, that feels better!' – and be able to work efficiently once more.

The type of food eaten should be chosen for its ability to release energy slowly but surely – good quality proteins like fish, free-range chicken, yoghurt, cottage cheese and tofu, beans and pulses like lentils and chickpeas, and also plenty of vegetables and whole grains to provide complex carbohydrates. It is good to aim for a balance of approximately one-third protein to two-thirds complex carbohydrates at every meal and every snack. You don't have to weigh it exactly – just roughly measuring portions to the palm of your hand will do – one palmful of chicken to two palmfuls of vegetables and/or grains. This advice is discussed in great detail in a book called *The Zone* by Dr Barry Sears which has already been mentioned in Chapter 6 – 'Stress'. It is based on a fairly recent understanding that providing this balance of fuel for our body's machinery is the way our biochemistry works best, and it certainly makes good scientific sense.

Says Dr Sears:

The rewards of increased energy, vitality and performance – in work, in play, in personal relationships – will amaze you. If this sounds like New Age jargon, it's not. It's the application of twenty-first century biotechnology solutions to a twentieth-century problem – how to increase the efficiency of the human body.

Try it for yourself and see if he's right!

The regulation of blood glucose (glucose is the simplest chemical form of sugar) is a constant balancing act. The aim is to provide energy to those cells of the body which need it (including the brain) and to make sure that unwanted glucose is not left circulating in the blood. If this balance is lost, both physical and mental well-being also become unbalanced.

Take careful note of the following Action Plan.

ACTION PLAN

1 It is better to eat five small meals a day than three large ones, but at least allow for snacks between breakfast, lunch and evening meal. Each meal and snack should contain a combination of protein (nuts, seeds, beans, yoghurt, cottage

cheese, egg, chicken, fish, tofu) and complex carbohydrate (vegetables – raw or lightly steamed, wholewheat crackers and pasta, rice and rice cakes, oats and oat cakes, etc.). Always aim for a balance of one-third protein to two-thirds complex carbohydrate.

2 Always eat breakfast and have a suitable snack at bedtime.

3 Avoid sugar, and foods containing sugar. Don't be tricked into thinking that demerara or raw cane sugar are good for you; they are not! Avoid honey, too – it is just another form of sugar, as also is malt. (And don't replace them with artificial sweeteners; they really are not good for you!)

4 Avoid refined grains (white flour, white rice, cornflour) because they are digested rapidly and so quickly enter the blood as glucose. Instead, eat whole grains – wholewheat flour, whole brown rice, maize meal (as opposed to refined cornflour) and various types of wholegrain pasta.

5 Avoid foods containing preservatives and chemical additives. This means avoiding all convenience foods – most of which will probably contain refined carbohydrates as well as harmful chemicals.

6 Keep fruit to a minimum – preferably avoid it. Avoid dried fruit completely because it is very high in fructose (natural fruit sugar). If you are on a candida diet, you are avoiding fruit in any case. It is worth pointing out that the candida diet is excellent for controlling blood glucose because it contains no sucrose, fructose or lactose!

7 Avoid fruit juice entirely.

8 Avoid all forms of alcohol.

9 Avoid tea and coffee, even if decaffeinated, because they still contain other stimulants. Also avoid cola drinks, chocolate drinks and Lucozade for the same reason.

10 Avoid painkillers and medications containing caffeine. Check the packet carefully before buying.

11 Determine to give up smoking.

12 Take regular exercise like walking – if you can. If you are suffering from severe CFS, you can forget this one for the time being!

13 Do all you can to avoid or deal with stress *(see Chapter 6 – 'Stress').*

14 Unless you can obtain or work out a tailor-made programme of supplements to meet your optimum daily requirements *(see Chapter 3 – 'Nutritional Deficiencies'),* try to take a good multivitamin/mineral supplement that includes vitamin B_3 50mg, vitamin B_5 50mg, zinc 15mg, manganese 10mg and chromium 200mcg. Also take at least 1 gram (1000mg) of vitamin C daily. This will support your liver in its production of Glucose Tolerance Factor, and also help to support your adrenals while things get back to normal.

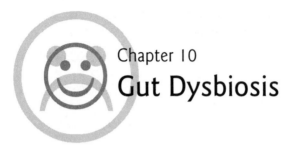

Chapter 10
Gut Dysbiosis

Working as a Nutrition Consultant and being involved with literally hundreds of CFS clients over the past several years, this piece of cargo is undoubtedly the one I have seen most frequently. I would go so far as to say that it can be found without exception in every ship that is sinking with CFS!

Dysbiosis means simply 'imbalance' so gut dysbiosis is an imbalance of micro-organisms in the intestines, often referred to as 'gut flora'. One of the most common causes of imbalanced gut flora is an overgrowth of *Candida albicans*, a yeast which lives inside each one of us but which under certain circumstances can spread and cause a wide variety of health problems, both physical and mental. This is such a common problem that it is necessary to talk about it at some length. Discussing CFS in his *Beat Fatigue Workbook*, Leon Chaitow says, 'What is certain is that concurrent infections such as candida (which very often accompanies ME/CFS) and hypoglycaemia (low blood sugar) must be considered and dealt with as first priorities if recovery is to be achieved.'

In fact, a severe case of candidiasis (an overgrowth of candida) is indistinguishable from CFS and the list of symptoms in the Introduction could be repeated word for word in a discussion on the effects of candida. Sometimes it is in fact the only piece of cargo which has overloaded the immune ship.

However, before candida entirely takes over this discussion on gut dysbiosis, let us first look at some other types of unfriendly microbes which might be causing chronic infection of the gut and also, if the gut wall is leaky, invading the bloodstream and causing systemic (by which is meant 'affecting the whole body') ill-health – placing an additional load on the liver and the immune system in the process.

You can suspect a possible parasitic infection if, besides suffering from chronic fatigue, you also have persistent intestinal problems and difficulty maintaining your body-weight – in other words, if you stay thin no matter how much you eat. Even this can be due to other things like gluten-intolerance but if this scenario is tied in with a history of being unwell ever since you had a tummy bug while visiting a country with a hot climate and a probable unsavoury water supply, there is very good cause to suspect that you might be carrying a parasite in your intestines.

Fortunately, parasites can usually be found in a stool specimen when it is investigated by a good laboratory procedure. Your doctor should be able to arrange this for you but, in case of difficulty, tests can be arranged by your nutritionist with Great Smokies laboratory in North Carolina, USA. These tests can be arranged in the UK through Health Interlink *(see Appendix B)*. Although it is possible to have a stool test which just looks for parasites, I usually take advantage of a special package run by Great Smokies because it includes two tests which together are extremely informative – a Comprehensive Digestive Stool Analysis and Comprehensive Parasitology. An Intestinal Permeability urine test is also very useful for showing if the gut wall has become leaky.

When any type of pathogenic bacteria is found in the CDSA, the laboratory report will include recommendations as to which pharmaceutical antibiotics and also which natural substances and herbs are most effective against that particular type of bacteria. If a parasite is found, your nutritionist will know how best to attack it with antifungal herbal supplements such as grapefruit seed extract, berberis and artemisia – unless, of course, you prefer to ask your doctor for an appropriate antibiotic, but this carries with it the risk of destroying your friendly bacteria which will possibly have been shown by the test to be low in any case.

It is often found that someone might have been carrying a parasite for years without it causing any problems until a second bad guy such as candida appears upon the scene, when they trigger each other into activity causing double-trouble.

I'd like to tell you about Jack whose mother brought him to see me when he was 14 years old and extremely unwell, weighing just under 35 kg (77 pounds). He had been off school for a year but had been ill all his life and treated with innumerable courses of antibiotics. He had been born in Hong Kong. I started by suspecting an overgrowth of candida and gave Jack a suitable nutritional programme to follow. He made some progress but not enough, so eventually I suggested the stool analysis. Jack was found to be carrying a parasite called *Dientamoeba fragilis*. Although it can sometimes cause no problems and is thought by some doctors to be a normal part of the intestinal environment, *Dientamoeba fragilis* is also known to lead to a variety of unpleasant symptoms including weight loss and fatigue. Jack's hospital specialist believed that the finding was meaningless but, undeterred, Jack's mother remained firm in her conviction that, having had the test, it was worth taking its findings seriously. I therefore prepared an appropriate nutritional plan of attack to vanquish *Dientamoeba fragilis*. Fourteen months later, Jack's weight had increased by 12.7 kg (28 pounds), he was back at school full-time with what his mother called 'oodles of energy', enjoying sport and doing very well with his studies. In a fitness test run by his school, he came fifth out of 150 boys!

Jack was left with a legacy of food sensitivities but as I write these are gradually being sorted out and overcome, and I have little doubt that in a couple of years he will be a very fit and healthy young man!

Other parasites are fairly common, too. I once collected (by eating salad on a Greek boat trip – be warned!) a parasite called *Blastocystis hominis* which gave me most uncomfortable abdominal pains. Fortunately, I had a rough idea what might be causing them so I did a stool test. When the results came back, I threw at *Blastocystis hominis* everything I knew from my nutritional expertise! The symptoms subsided and have never recurred.

So, having given some thought to parasites and intestinal bacteria, let's now turn to what is probably the biggest and boldest bad guy of them all, the yeast *Candida albicans*! The name means 'sweet and white', suggesting something delicate and pure – which could not be further from the truth. *Candida albicans* is a minute microbe, a yeast, which can afflict us with innumerable symptoms, both physical and mental, many of which mimic other diseases and are therefore frequently misdiagnosed. Its dark and devious character is the very opposite of what its name implies!

Many who suffer at the hands of this microbe see candida as a personal enemy, a dark invader who threatens to overwhelm them and against whom they must engage in long and determined warfare. The only certain way to victory is to understand the enemy's tactics and take the offensive with all guns blazing. This enemy will lose no opportunity to retake lost ground, so the battle must be unrelenting until at last it is won – and even then there is the danger of a false treaty, when you think the enemy is under control but it is in fact just biding its time before making another onslaught!

The imagery of warfare is strengthened by the fact that thriving candida takes on a fungal form, and the ecological function of a fungus is to recycle organic material. To candida, the human body is a pile of organic material and, given half a chance, it will take advantage of a depressed immune system or a deficiency of friendly bacteria in the intestines and start to recycle *us!* Though possibly not a fight to the death, the battle is certainly on for quality of life. Candida multiplies, migrates and releases toxins, causing bowel problems, allergy, hormonal problems, skin complaints, joint and muscle pain, thrush, infections, fatigue and emotional disorders – to name but a few! It is little wonder that candida sufferers frequently say they feel ill all over.

The battle starts in our intestines, where we each carry about 1.75 kg (4 pounds) of microbes. When we are healthy, these little organisms are divided into about 80 per cent 'good guys' and 20 per cent potential 'bad guys', each with a part to play in our internal ecology. The bad guys are actually quite harmless and even useful while they stay within their '20 per cent' boundary, but trouble begins when they overgrow. *Candida albicans* is one of these potential bad guys and unfortunately many things are happening in this day and age which encourage it to spread and become aggressive.

If you were to look at candida through a fairly powerful microscope, you would see a small white speck. In fact it is a spore, rather like a tiny mushroom. Once it is strong in numbers, however, it is able to change to a fungal form, where it puts out root-like structures called mycelia. Now if you look through a microscope, you will see something that looks for all the world like mould that is growing on an old piece of bread; it is now in a form where it is able to invade the body's tissues and cause a fungal infection.

The situation is largely man-made. Candida is a yeast, and yeasts thrive on sugar, as anyone will know who has ever made bread, beer or wine. The process is started by placing sugar and yeast together and leaving them in a warm place to ferment. As well as stirring sugar into tea and coffee, we consume it in vast amounts in most pre-packaged foods because its preservative properties ensure a longer shelf-life and its sweet taste guarantees its customer-appeal. Remember, it is reckoned that the majority of people today eat more than their own body-weight in sugar every single year! *(see Chapter 3 – 'Nutritional deficiencies')*. Another factor which adds to the body's sugar load is that refined grains like white flour and white rice break down to glucose once digested much more quickly than whole grains, so much of our modern-day diet is encouraging bad guys to flourish.

At the same time as all this, the number of good guys we carry is often being reduced by the indiscriminate use of antibiotics. Many people expect their doctor to prescribe antibiotics for any type of infection, whether it has been caused by bacteria or a virus. In fact, antibiotics are not effective against viruses and, even when used appropriately (for instance, for secondary bacterial infection following a virus infection), these powerful drugs, which so often save lives, not only kill the bug which has made you ill but also destroy your friendly bacteria, which allows thriving yeasts more room in which to spread. Besides all the antibiotics which are medically prescribed, we also receive residues of them in meat and dairy products because many animals are given antibiotics by their breeders purely as a preventative measure to keep them healthy for market – a good reason for buying organic meat, if you can.

Another cause of overgrowths of candida is the use of steroids, and this includes the contraceptive pill and hormone treatments which, among other things, suppress the body's immune response in the same way as all other forms of steroid treatment. It is fairly common to find young women with severe problems of candida or CFS who have been on the Pill since the age of 13 because they had painful periods. It is becoming increasingly common to find older women suffering with similar health problems after being on HRT (hormone replacement therapy). Sometimes it has taken several years for their health to be affected, sometimes it happens quite quickly. Seldom has an initial attempt been made to try to improve their menopausal symptoms through nutritional means, yet in the vast majority of cases this is all that is needed, even as a preventative measure against osteoporosis – especially if adequate load-bearing exercise can be taken because this enhances bone density.

Asthma sufferers who are prescribed steroid inhalers frequently develop thrush infections of the mouth and throat, and eczema sufferers using steroid creams often develop problems of weakened immunity including an increase in allergy. One of the first situations to suffer is the balance of bacteria in the intestines, as the immune system grows too weak to hold back invaders. Another factor with regard to steroid treatments is that, according to Elizabeth Lipski in her book *Digestive Wellness*, they provide excellent nourishment for fungi, and therefore for candida in its fungal form.

Another major reason why so many people are suffering from symptoms related to yeast infection is that we have a generation which to a large extent was not breast-fed, and breast milk should ensure that a baby starts life with a healthy balance of friendly intestinal bacteria. I say this with some reservation because of course the quality of breast-milk depends on the mother's nutritional status and also upon pollution factors. It has been claimed that *all* human breast-milk world-wide, whether in Western urban cities or South American jungles, is now contaminated with pesticides and other environmental toxins which damage the friendly bacteria in a baby's intestines. The situation has deteriorated so badly that the balance of microbes in the intestines of today's breast-fed baby is reckoned to be the same as that of a bottle-fed baby 40 years ago! Even so, breast-milk contains caprylic acid, an antifungal substance which is otherwise found in coconuts, and this means that breast-fed babies do obtain a degree of protection against an overgrowth of yeast in their bodies, an advantage which bottle-fed babies don't have.

So, the foregoing factors and others besides mean that our generation has a problem which is fast becoming epidemic, so it is quite surprising that many doctors still appear to be unaware of it. Yet in researching for a dissertation on candida which I wrote in my third year of training, I found a weighty medical textbook entitled, *Candida and Candidosis* by Professor F.C. Odds (now sadly out of print – presumably through lack of interest), which contained well over 5,000 medical references to the condition.

So what happens when the yeast in our intestines gets out of control? In its fungal form it can travel to any part of the body and establish a colony just wherever it chooses! It particularly seems to make a beeline for any traumatized tissue in the body (old injuries, operation areas, arthritic joints), although I have only anecdotal evidence for this. As it burrows through tissues, it can cause problems anywhere in the body – perhaps in the vagina (causing irritation, soreness or discharge), the urinary tract (causing kidney infections and cystitis), the sinuses, ears, throat or bronchial passages (causing chronic respiratory infections), the skin (causing acne, eczema and psoriasis), muscles (causing weakness, tremor, numbness, tingling or even paralysis), or joints (causing stiffness, pain and swelling).

Because the root of yeast overgrowth is in the colon, diarrhoea or constipation (or both!) and abdominal pain are frequently experienced, so that very many people with candidiasis have been diagnosed as having irritable bowel syndrome or colitis – both of which are simply descriptive terms that don't identify the cause. Bloating and wind are very common indeed as the imbalance of bacteria causes fermentation in the intestines. From the colon, the fungus will often travel downwards (causing an itchy bottom or painful spasm in the anus); and it will also migrate upwards (causing nausea and pain in the stomach and then soreness and pain of the oesophagus, throat and mouth).

In women, a common effect of candida is to block the efficient working of their hormones. Candida has receptor sites in its cell membranes which accept hormones, thus preventing them from reaching their proper destination. In addition, candida exactly fits the receptor sites which are waiting for the hormones, so this is a second way in which hormone function is blocked. (This information was published in *Science* magazine in 1984 by David Feldman, in an article entitled, 'Steroid Hormone Systems Found in Yeast'.) Because candida also triggers auto-immune processes, creating antibodies to the body's own hormones, symptoms increase cyclically with the menstrual cycle, regularly flaring up before or after a period. (Another effect of this hormonal interaction is that enormous numbers of women develop thrush during their nine months of pregnancy.) It would therefore appear that premenstrual symptoms might not be due entirely to a hormonal imbalance (which you can expect to be corrected in any case as your nutritional status improves), but that they are at least in part due to an increase in candida activity. Even infertility can be helped by bringing candida under control and improving nutritional status, and I am delighted to have seen several clients, previously infertile, conceive without difficulty when these situations have been tackled and dealt with.

Once pregnant, it is not a good idea to wage full warfare against candida until after the baby has been born and weaned. This is because dead candida releases a great many toxins into the mother's bloodstream, which obviously does not provide a healthy environment for the baby, neither at a later stage would you want to risk the toxins entering the baby through the breast milk. However, it is certainly worth keeping to an anti-candida diet during pregnancy and while breast-feeding, and also taking a good supplement programme to supply levels of nutrients which not only will help to boost immunity but will also be beneficial for the baby. With these measures, I have often seen symptoms improve during pregnancy, even though candida activity would normally increase at this time. However, as soon as breast-feeding has stopped, it is obviously a good idea to ensure that candida is fully under control by taking all the necessary steps as described in the following chapter.

Another situation which strongly displays the link between hormones and candida is endometriosis; here again, marked improvements can sometimes be achieved by following the full anti-candida programme. A book called *Overcoming Endometriosis* (Arlington Books, 1988) included one contribution entitled, 'Endometriosis and Yeast: A New Connection' and another entitled, 'Endometriosis and Candidiasis: More Startling Connections'.

Men are just as susceptible to candidiasis as women but, partly because candida and female hormones so strongly interact and also because women have more areas where candida can thrive, the condition is possibly not quite so common in men. In addition to symptoms which are common to both sexes, women may develop an abnormal menstrual cycle, pre-menstrual tension, violent mood swings, periods which are painful or heavy, and countless numbers suffer from chronic vaginal thrush. In men, the most common symptoms are abdominal bloating, wind and either constipation or diarrhoea, but they also may have aches and pains in muscles and joints, depression, anxiety, bad temper and sensitivities to food and chemicals. It is possible for candida to be transmitted through sexual contact, and so thrush can be passed back and forth between partners, quite often without realizing it if the effects are mainly systemic.

If a mother is suffering from vaginal thrush at the time of giving birth (which is quite likely to happen because the hormonal changes in pregnancy encourage candida to thrive – especially if she has previously taken the Pill), the baby will almost certainly pick it up at the very start of life on its journey through the birth canal. While it is inside the womb, a baby's gut is completely sterile. In a healthy state of affairs, the first microbes to enter his intestines will be friendly bacteria supplied in his mother's breast milk. The poor infant whose intestines are populated with unfriendly yeasts even before he has had a chance to suck his first milk is probably going to suffer from oral thrush, severe nappy rash and colic in his early weeks, and this quite often will lead to problems of a weakened immune system, which in turn will lead to ear infections, tonsillitis and eczema which will be treated with antibiotics and steroid creams, which will encourage the candida in his intestines to flourish even more. In line with the old nursery rhyme, this is the house that candida built! The unhealthy infant is all set to become a chronically ill adult.

To start with, candida might give rise to just a few symptoms which you consider to be minor problems that almost everyone has to put up with – possibly indigestion, intestinal gas and bloating, depression, PMT, a tendency to catch colds and some occasional rectal or vaginal irritation. It then progresses to a stage where a whole host of different symptoms develop but unfortunately there is often nothing to be seen, and as the condition is incredibly difficult to diagnose by any kind of test, you continue to think that these symptoms are somehow what life is about. Since every person has *some* candida, many tests will give a positive result yet it seems that quite a few medical practitioners discount this as being 'normal', without investigating the *level* of candida present. This is certainly often the case with vaginal swabs which are given a 'Normal' test result even though the poor woman is climbing the wall with inflammation and irritation and is obviously also affected by candida all over her body!

Of the various laboratory tests for candida that are available, many of them have shortcomings. An interesting discussion of testing techniques can be found in *Optimal Wellness*, by Dr Ralph Golan, who summarizes the situation by saying that in general, an assessment of symptoms and history usually provides as valuable information about his patients as laboratory tests. Why is testing not reliable? One reason is that stool cultures can be misleading because, if yeast is in its fungal form, most of the cells will be physically attached or will have burrowed into the intestinal lining, so that a stool culture can only detect cells which have literally broken off – of which maybe there are none. Neither can an internal endoscopy examination with a camera be considered foolproof because candida does not colonize the gut in a uniform fashion but forms clusters and nests and hides itself away in any pockets it can find.

Blood tests which look for candida antibodies can also be misleading unless all types of antibody are investigated – IgA, IgE, IgG and IgM –because, for instance, finding high levels of candida IgG antibodies does not necessarily mean a current overgrowth of yeast, simply that there was one once! High IgE might mean an allergy to yeast rather than an overgrowth of it, and even IgM antibodies that measure recent infections are not necessarily going to be able to detect yeast in the intestinal tract at a stage when yeast might not yet have invaded the bloodstream. In fact, one intensive study reported by Dr William Shaw in his book, *Biological Treatments for Autism and PDD*, showed a very high incidence of false negatives in blood cultures of children who later died. Autopsies showed that they actually had yeast invasion of various body organs, including liver, heart and brain, yet only 17 per cent of their blood samples had tested positive for yeast even though they had been tested an average of 10 times.

Possibly one of the most reliable tests for detecting elevated levels of yeast in the body is an organic acid urine test. It looks for by-products of yeast and fungi which have been produced in the intestinal tract and then absorbed into the bloodstream and eventually found their way into the urine. This test is undertaken by an American laboratory called Great Plains, based in Kansas (available through practitioners in the UK and elsewhere via Health Interlink – *see Appendix B*). Although certainly a useful test, it is expensive and I have used it on only a very few occasions when the client has felt he needed some positive proof of his candida diagnosis.

None of these tests mentioned are widely used by medical practitioners and so very often someone who is suffering from a whole spectrum of candida-related problems also has to suffer the loneliness of being misdiagnosed and misunderstood and the indignity of being labelled a hypochondriac – situations well-known to many sufferers of CFS. Being told that your pain is 'all in your mind' never helped anyone, and, in any case, where is the help for the mind?

Obviously, in considering whether to launch an attack against candida, it is very important to ensure that the enemy is correctly identified. So, without the help of a laboratory test, how can this be done? Before giving nutritional advice, I ensure that my clients have had all the medical tests which their doctors have considered necessary and made available. If no cause for their problems has been found, a suitable questionnaire can then help to ascertain the presence or severity of an overgrowth of candida – and is usually all that is needed. For a long time I used one which had been devised by Dr William Crook, author of *The Yeast Connection*; now I have devised one myself and you will find it at the back of this book *(Appendix A)*. If it shows a high score (or even one that is slightly raised), and if doctors have failed to make any other diagnosis, it makes sense to embark on an anti-candida campaign. The questionnaire provides a comprehensive list of signs and symptoms that are commonly associated with an overgrowth of candida. My own story of lifelong health problems due to candida is written in Chapter 16 of this book, where many of its effects are described from personal and bitter experience!

Candida in its fungal form releases a great many toxins (according to Professor Odds, no less than 79 have been identified!) which escape through the leaky gut wall created by candida roots and, besides causing physical symptoms like muscular aches, lack of energy, weakness and fatigue, they also cause mental or emotional symptoms – foggy head, feelings of unreality, depression, anxiety, irritability, loss of memory, lack of concentration, inability to make decisions. Such symptoms can vary from being slight and occasional right through to being totally incapacitating and seemingly unending.

In addition to all this, the immune system has an enormous fight on its hands as it tries to hold back invading candida, and the body becomes increasingly unable to fight off any other invaders when they appear, thus allowing allergies and infections to take hold more easily. The regularity with which candida is seen in cases of CFS suggests that when a particular virus (causing, for instance, glandular fever or flu) first attempted to launch its attack, the body was unable to fight it off because the immune system was already too busy and exhausted from trying to cope with candida. Once again, it's the picture of the overloaded cargo ship.

The vast majority of CFS sufferers that I come across had initially been treated with antibiotics for the infection they were fighting, with the outcome that their illness became chronic instead of being simply a short-term attack. This is because antibiotics had depleted their colonies of friendly bacteria, allowing bad guys like candida to overgrow and place even more of a load on the immune system. I was recently delighted to see in my local surgery a leaflet entitled, 'Antibiotics – Who Needs Them?', an attempt by the medical profession to re-educate the public in their understanding and expectation of antibiotics. Hopefully, the tide has begun to turn.

Food allergy is very common in candida sufferers. When candida in its fungal form penetrates the intestinal wall, it leaves it porous, as described in Chapter 2 – 'Allergy'. In this situation, the immune system treats the arrival of a food particle as an enemy instead of a friend, and calls out all its troops to deal with it, resulting in an 'allergic' or sensitivity reaction. In future, each time that particular food comes into the body, it is recognized by the troops and dealt with in the same way, and we are left with sensitivity to it. An intestinal wall which has become very porous paves the way for a great many 'food allergies' in some people, leaving them desperately short of foods they can eat without feeling ill.

Inhaled allergens also become a problem. Things like paint and household cleaners often create a nightmare of symptoms, both physical and mental. Domestic gas and petrol fumes do the same. Some people experience a horrendous reaction to perfumes or after-shave, which sadly plays havoc with any social life they might still manage to enjoy! Reactions to local anaesthetics have even more dire consequences, as I found to my cost when for 17 years I had to have all my dentistry without an injection!

Eventually, after years of sickness, I realized that I had managed to put together a four-point plan which has since been effective in restoring the health of countless other lives besides my own. Later, when I trained for three years at the Institute for Optimum Nutrition in London, I came to understand the biochemical reasons for its effectiveness. In the next chapter, I give details of this Four-Point Plan – the Action Plan for this particular piece of cargo.

We cannot put *all* the blame on candida for ruining our lives; in this day and age we are giving it every encouragement and opportunity to do so. The first stage in fighting back is therefore to start taking personal responsibility for our own health.

ACTION PLAN

Read Part Two!

Part ②

Beat Candida

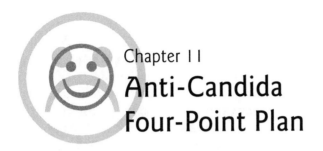

Chapter 11

Anti-Candida Four-Point Plan

Since an overgrowth of *Candida albicans* has been a factor in every single case of CFS that I have come across, it is vital to do everything possible to ensure that it is brought fully under control, and this will not be achieved unless, as I have said before, it is attacked with all guns blazing. Omitting just one part of the four-point plan, or failing to keep strictly to the diet, is sufficient cause to lose the battle, whereas with understanding, determination and perseverance, the battle can most certainly be won!

Outlined below is the four-point plan which brought victory in my own life and, since then, in the lives of thousands of others:

1 Anti-candida diet.
2 Personal supplement programme.
3 Antifungal supplements.
4 Probiotics – the 'good guys'.

I The Anti-Candida Diet

The aim of the diet is to starve overgrowths of candida to death! Since sugar encourages and activates yeast, all forms of sugar must be strictly avoided – not just sucrose (packet sugar, whether white or brown), but also lactose (in milk), fructose (in fruit and honey), glucose and dextrose (both of which are often listed as ingredients) and malt. Some authors and practitioners allow fruit to be reintroduced after the first few weeks, but I have never seen candida brought *fully* under control whilst any fruit is allowed at all. Refined carbohydrates add to the glucose load so it is essential to use only whole grain wheatflour, whole grain brown rice, maize meal instead of refined cornflour, etc. Other substances to be avoided are yeast (yeasted bread, gravy mixes, spreads), fermented products (alcohol, vinegar), mould (cheese, mushrooms), and stimulants (tea, coffee). (Incidentally, this is a sidetrack but did you know that you can often find three or more different types of sugar listed among ingredients on a packet? UK food laws state that ingredients should be listed in descending order of amounts, so if you put in three different types of sugar each at a fairly low level, e.g. lactose, dextrose and fructose, you are not actually showing the total sugar content because that would put it top of the list of ingredients! Look for this on some labels next time you are in your supermarket.)

A positive attitude to the diet is essential, and I wrote the *Beat Candida Cookbook* to show that mealtimes can still be enjoyable. The book includes ideas for two weeks' menus together with shopping lists, and it contains over 300 recipes, each of which is given a star rating based on the energy required to prepare it, a coding system which many people have said they appreciate. One-star recipes (*) involve little more than opening a tin and a packet and perhaps putting something in the oven, two star recipes (**) require a little more energy for mixing or chopping, and three-star recipes (***) take more preparation so can be attempted when you are feeling stronger, and they may be served at a dinner party to guests who will be quite unaware that they are eating an anti-candida starter, main course and dessert! The anti-candida diet guidelines are included now as Chapter 17, sample menus for a week are included as Chapter 18, and recipes to go with the menus may be found in Chapter 19.

A craving for candida's favourite foods is frequently experienced, and at these times steely determination is needed to keep to the diet. However, if temptation threatens to win the day, an amino acid supplement called L-Glutamine can help to damp down a craving for sweet foods or alcohol. Motivation is encouraged by a clear understanding of what is happening. Even when candida-related symptoms have completely disappeared, the diet should be maintained for a further year in order to consolidate the newly-corrected balance of intestinal microbes, otherwise known as 'gut flora'.

After being deprived of all forms of sugar for a while, a 'sweet tooth' can no longer survive. We were not born with it so if it is not encouraged it will actually go away, making it much easier to stay on a sugar-free diet which of course will help to maintain good health in the future, even when candida is fully under control.

It is my fervent hope that the anti-candida diet will be seen as an opportunity to learn how to *enjoy* eating healthily, because this will help to lay a foundation for continued good health in years to come. Hopefully no-one, once cured of yeast infection, will ever again have the slightest desire to return to eating the junk foods and sugar-laden products which almost certainly helped to make them ill in the first place!

There is one very big bonus which is frequently experienced by overweight people when they start on the anti-candida diet – they lose weight, quickly and easily! This has nothing to do with the fact that their food intake has been reduced, because it hasn't; they can eat as much as they like of the foods which are allowed. The reason for this pleasing weight-loss is that the body has been able to offload some unwanted fluid, which had previously been retained to reduce the impact of yeasty foods. The same would apply to almost any other food to which there was a sensitivity, and an immune system which has become hypersensitive to overgrowths of yeast in the body will mount a reaction when confronted with yeast in the diet. As part of this reaction, fluid is retained, but when yeasty foods are avoided, the fluid comes away – at a much faster rate than it is possible to burn up fat. I had one very overweight client who lost 38 kg (84 pounds or 6 stone) in six months, and she said it had been the easiest thing in the world, because she never once had to feel hungry.

The other side of the same coin, however, is that sometimes people who are of average weight, or even underweight, will also lose some fluid when they start to follow the anti-candida diet. If the fluid is there, it needs to come away, and it indicates that some of the weight they previously carried, even if they were thin, was not in fact due to healthy body tissue. Once the fluid has been offloaded, weight-loss will normally stabilize. In due course, as all the systems start to work more efficiently by following a nutritional regime and as appropriate exercise can be built into the lifestyle, each person's weight will become whatever is healthy for their sex, age, height and bone structure. Look after your health, and your weight will look after itself!

2 Personal Supplement Programme

As a student at the Institute for Optimum Nutrition, I was taught the basic concept of 'biochemical individuality'. This simply means that each of us has an individual nutritional status, reflecting strengths and weaknesses of the immune system, etc., which is as unique as our finger-prints, so that we each require levels and balances of vitamins and minerals which are specific to our personal needs.

I also learned to use a Nutrition Programme Questionnaire to assess each person's nutritional requirements through an analysis of their symptoms and diet. I discovered that buying a pot of vitamins from a health-food store might possibly turn out to be a complete waste of money unless the assistant knew a thing or two and could also provide some responsible advice. It is simply not possible for the contents of one particular multivitamin and mineral supplement to meet the exact requirements of every person who buys it!

Our inherited tendencies, medical history, lifestyle and diet all make us biochemical individuals, which means that each person requires a tailor-made programme of supplements which will meet his own specific needs at any given time and so ensure that biochemical imbalances and deficiencies are corrected by regulating the body's nutritional status. In this way, all the body systems, including the immune system, may be encouraged to function with the greatest possible efficiency.

A supplement programme of vitamins, minerals, essential fatty acids and sometimes amino acids must be devised to help correct imbalances in glucose tolerance, hormonal status and histamine levels. Appropriate nutrients are also needed to detoxify the body of pollutants, help improve stress reactions and encourage a healthy heart and arteries. In addition, it is obviously extremely important to support the immune system in as many ways as possible in order, among other things, to help it fight back at encroaching colonies of candida. This has been discussed in more detail in Chapter 3 – 'Nutritional Deficiencies', where I said that Patrick Holford in his book, *Optimum Nutrition*, gives helpful guidelines on how you can calculate your own supplement requirements. Otherwise, of course, a trained nutritionist will do it for you.

Time and again I am impressed by the improvement in a client's health when I review their nutritional status after they have been on therapeutic levels of nutrients for a period of three months. This allows time for the nutrients to get into the body and do their work and means that the supplement programme may then be pruned down to meet their new optimum level of nutritional requirements. Eventually, it will be cut right down to maintenance levels when this is all that is required to keep their body functioning at its best.

Even this ongoing programme should be tailor-made to take into account specific situations like the presence of mercury in amalgam fillings and, in a post-menopausal woman, the right levels and proportions of nutrients to guard against the possibility of developing brittle bones. This is a far more natural approach than hormone replacement therapy which not only may have hazardous side-effects but almost certainly will depress the immune system, due to its steroid action.

In an otherwise carefully-calculated programme of nutrients, vitamin C may be taken to bowel tolerance levels to rid the body of candida toxins, just as when fighting an infection or an allergy. It is taken at intervals throughout the day until you have a loose bowel motion, and then you stop. Next day, you do the same thing but you will probably find that less vitamin C is needed to achieve the same result. When the body is fighting infection or toxins, its tissues will soak up vitamin C just like a sponge, but eventually it will eliminate through the bowel any that is surplus to requirements, hence the loose stools. Of course, vitamin C should never be taken on its own. Make sure that you also take a comprehensive programme of the other vitamins and minerals, as just described *(and see Chapter 3 – 'Nutritional Deficiencies')*.

3 Antifungal Supplements

One of the most useful antifungal agents is caprylic acid, a fatty acid which occurs naturally in coconuts. It is far less toxic than any pharmaceutical antifungal drug, and it has a great advantage in that it does not adversely affect the friendly microbes. Being a natural fatty acid, it is reasonably well able to be absorbed through the gut wall, but its primary battle-ground is in the intestines. Taken as a combination of calcium caprylate and magnesium caprylate, it survives digestive processes and is able to reach the colon. For reasons which I shall explain in Chapter 12 – 'Die-off!', it is essential to start with a low level of antifungal supplements and build up gradually.

Certain herbs like oregano, cloves and artemisia produce oils which also have effective antifungal properties, and because their chemical structure is smaller than that of caprylic acid, they are even better able to be absorbed through the gut wall. A supplement containing these herbal oils is therefore useful for reaching parts of the body where candida has colonized outside the digestive tract. However, since the root of an overgrowth of candida is always in the colon, I find that caprylic acid is usually the better supplement to start with and possibly it is the only one which will be needed, but that remains to be seen. In the first place, allow caprylic acid to do all it can in bringing candida under control in the intestines; after that, if necessary, we can mount an attack in outlying areas where candida has taken up residence by changing to the herbal oil product which has greater systemic activity.

If other types of bad guy besides candida are suspected, or have been confirmed by a stool test or parasitology investigation, there are other herbs which have a more broad-spectrum effect. Grapefruit seed extract, artemisia, golden seal, berberis and uva ursi are some of the herbs which have broad-spectrum properties, making them useful against a wide range of undesirable microbes and parasites but with the advantage that they do not disturb the friendly bacteria. This makes them preferable to garlic which, in my experience, is so effective against a wide range of micro-organisms that it also can destroy the good guys and should therefore be regarded with as much caution as an antibiotic drug. However, this applies mainly to garlic supplements and it is unlikely that a *small* amount of garlic used for flavouring your food will cause very much of a problem.

A liquid antifungal product can be obtained which has a very different approach. It introduces oxygen to the tissues in the form of hyperoxygenated sodium ions on the principle that oxygen is antagonistic to yeast organisms, and in particular to *Candida albicans*. It is not the same as hydrogen peroxide, which has a different chemical structure. When diluted, it is particularly useful as a mouthwash for oral thrush, as a gargle for fungal throat conditions and as a nasal douche for congested sinuses, a condition which frequently leads to dizziness and spaced-out feelings. My advice for doing this is to dilute 2 drops in 2 table-spoons of tepid water, pour half into the palm of one hand, put your nose down into it and sniff it up one nostril. Keep sniffing to hold the liquid in your nasal passages for as long as possible. (You'll need plenty of tissues around to mop yourself up!) Then repeat with the other hand and the other nostril. This antifungal liquid may also be applied undiluted to fungal toe-nails.

Propolis is another natural substance which, according to research carried out in 1976 at the University of Bratislava, is remarkably effective for all fungal infections of the skin and body. It should be taken as an alcohol-free tincture, diluted and – if taken internally – increased gradually as with any other type of antifungal. Its slightly anaesthetic effect can be most soothing for oral thrush, besides having good antifungal and antibacterial properties. Propolis is made by bees to coat the inside of the hive, which is apparently the most sterile environment to be found in nature! It is certainly worth trying in the initial stage of an infection in the hope that you might be able to avoid the need for an antibiotic.

Aloe vera is gently antifungal and is a refreshing mouthwash or gargle as well as an aid to digestion. It can be used as an overnight denture soak, making it preferable to products which are not specifically antifungal. Dentures can be an ongoing source of candida re-infection. One difficulty with aloe vera, whether as juice or gel, is that it is difficult to find a product which contains no citric acid. By this I don't just mean natural lemon juice, I mean the commercially-produced form of citric acid which is a derivative of yeast and should therefore be avoided.

Any antifungal substance should be used with caution and special care should be taken when using two at the same time, as for instance when you are already taking caprylic acid and then decide to try propolis to help your painful gums. This is because the effect of destroying too much candida too quickly can be quite devastating, as I shall explain shortly. The best thing in these circumstances, if you have a symptom requiring propolis, is to have a temporary break from caprylic acid.

Tea tree oil is another antifungal substance which, as a cream, may be used for fungal skin conditions like acne, eczema, psoriasis or athlete's foot, and also for vaginal thrush and rectal soreness or irritation. Although skin complaints like eczema are often due to an unsuspected food allergy, they are also frequently fungal in origin and will respond to an anti-candida regime. However, they usually seem to get worse before they get better, as fungal toxins are pushed to the surface of the body. You do need to be patient in waiting for fungal skin conditions to clear because although the balance of microbes on the surface of the skin reflects the balance in the intestines, it is three months behind. In other words, you have to concentrate the attack on intestinal candida first, and then patiently wait another three months for your skin to clear – although herbal creams like tea tree (antifungal), chickweed (for irritation), marigold (for cracks) or propolis salve (for reducing inflammation) can help to alleviate conditions like eczema, psoriasis or acne while you are waiting.

With careful experimentation, the most suitable antifungal products can soon be found and put to good use, but first it is important that you should read Chapter 12 so that you understand about die-off reaction, and you need to take special note of the advice in that chapter on how to start by taking just low levels of antifungals and building them up gradually.

4 Probiotics – the 'Good Guys'

Supplements are needed to carry beneficial bacteria into the intestines and re-establish a healthy colony of gut flora. I once read an article by an American author where he referred to this process as 're-florestation', which I think is a lovely word! The role of these 'good guys' is to increase acidity and to hold back the 'bad guys'. Tissues densely covered with beneficial organisms provide an effective blocking mechanism against invaders.

Lactobacillus acidophilus is the major colonizer of the small intestine and *Bifidobacterium bifidum* inhabits the vagina and the large intestine, where it produces significant amounts of B vitamins for use in the body. Other helpful bacteria are *Lactobacillus bulgaricus* and *Streptococcus thermophilus*. These friendly bacteria are contained in yoghurt which is therefore helpful, provided there is no intolerance to dairy foods. In yoghurt, the lactose content of milk has largely been converted into lactic acid by enzyme-producing bacteria, which accounts for the sharpness of its taste. However, to ensure safe passage of friendly bacteria through the gastric juices, it is necessary to take them in a capsule containing large numbers of good guys freeze-dried in powder form. Two capsules should be taken daily, one at breakfast and one at supper, but this may be increased to six capsules daily or even more in cases of diarrhoea or following an unavoidable course of antibiotics, which further deplete the all-important beneficial bacteria.

Care should be taken that the supplements used contain both *L. acidophilus* and *Bifidobacterium* and supply a total of at least four billion viable cells per daily dose. The product should clearly show its expiry date and the manufacturer should be prepared to supply you with full information. In an independent analysis of 22 commercially-available products carried out by the University of Wales, only three came up to specified standards and several brands fell short even of their own stated specifications!

An absorbent cream taking lactic acid into vaginal tissue is a beneficial aid for thrush by creating an acidic environment which discourages the growth of yeast in the area. This can be most soothing and helpful while the four-point plan is getting to grips with the intestinal situation that underlies the problem. Vaginal thrush will almost certainly not be completely overcome until the balance of bacteria in the intestines has been corrected, but it is great to have help available in the meantime! It is also a good idea for both sexual partners to use this type of cream, to reduce the risk of persistent cross-infection. Sometimes it is helpful to use a natural antifungal cream (like one containing tea tree oil) in the morning, and the lactic acid cream at night, providing a two-pronged approach.

5 Support – the Fifth Point in the Four-Point Plan!

Each of the points in the four-point plan is essential in the fight against candida. Omitting any one of them will end in failure. However, there is also a fifth point which is just as vital, and that is SUPPORT.

Anyone entering the candida war zone will almost certainly find themselves in a minefield of problems. Confusion and depression abound, and someone is needed who can look at the situation objectively, discern what is happening and point the way forward. This is part of the role of an effective nutritionist.

You also need to gather your home team around you! Explain your nutritional regime to your family and friends, tell them what to expect from die-off reaction and ask them to stand with you and encourage you through it whenever it happens. Help them to understand your 'strange' new way of eating so that they don't make mistakes in preparing your food – or worse, try to tempt you to stray from the diet. With friends like that, who needs enemies? Try to get each friend and family member to be on your side and cheer you on, so that you can be certain of plenty of strong support at those times when you most need it.

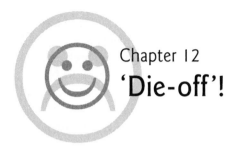

Chapter 12
'Die-off'!

I have already said that thriving candida releases a minimum of 79 known toxins. Dead candida releases even more. This can lead to symptoms which seem like a flare-up of any of your old problems (for instance, sore throat, thrush, painful joints, eczema) because candida is now dying in the areas where it had been living, so these are the places where it releases extra toxins and makes you aware of the effects.

It can also lead to flu-like symptoms, because large numbers of toxins circulating in the bloodstream can cause aching muscles, fuzzy head, depression, anxiety, irritability and diarrhoea. In fact, they can do almost anything to your tummy, reversing previous bowel habits and increasing nausea, bloating and wind. Perhaps worst of all, they might make you feel severely anxious or depressed.

This unpleasant situation is known as 'die-off reaction' (or more formally as 'Herxheimer's reaction') and during these times you need the courage of your convictions that you are only experiencing these symptoms because your overgrowth of yeast is being brought under control which means you are on the way to getting well – no matter how poorly you feel!

There is quite a lot that can be done to regulate and control the severity of die-off reaction, but even so you need to know in advance that the going might get tough at times. A large part of my working week is taken up with providing 'back-up' support which is offered for three months following each consultation, to encourage clients to contact me with any questions or problems which might arise.

Die-off needs to be recognized as a last-ditch deception by the enemy because the very presence of the symptoms means that candida is being wiped out and that victory is imminent.

Severe die-off usually indicates that candida is being destroyed faster than the body can eliminate the extra toxins; it can therefore be avoided by reducing antifungal supplements in order to allow the body time to offload the backlog of toxins. The art of the exercise is to destroy candida slowly but surely, and initial die-off will probably be triggered by the diet (as candida is starved to death) and by vitamins and minerals (as they boost the immune system to start fighting back). These first two points of the four-point plan often cause as much die-off reaction as most people want to cope with, so antifungal agents should not be added to the regime until this phase is over.

By the end of a month on the diet and tailor-made supplement programme, the majority of people are able to say that they feel better than they have for a very long time! Then is the time to add caprylic acid or other antifungals together with acidophilus supplements. Sometimes it takes longer than a month to reach this stage, depending on the situation, but it is certain to come in due course.

Taking ground slowly is still the surest method of attack. Most people on caprylic acid can start by tolerating a medium-strength capsule, 400 mg once daily, without too much difficulty. If, after five days, they are not battling with die-off symptoms, the dose may be increased to 400 mg twice daily, and so on up to six capsules daily. After this, they can transfer to 680 mg three times daily and increase again if necessary.

However, the climb-up is seldom straightforward as at any stage there might come a surge of die-off reaction, in which case it would be foolish to make matters worse by increasing the level of antifungals. You therefore either remain at the same level for longer than five days, or you drop back to a lower level until die-off symptoms have subsided. Then you start to increase again. Sometimes, if die-off symptoms are really unpleasant, I advise a complete break from antifungals for up to a month, to allow time for the body to offload the backlog of toxins. After that, it is usually easier to move forward again with antifungals. Such a break should not be regarded as a setback, but simply as a necessary part of the process. Drinking plenty of fluid and taking good levels of vitamin C, as already discussed, will speed up detoxification. If a high level of caprylic acid has been taken and it appears to have achieved as much as it can yet some symptoms still persist, it might be necessary to transfer to another type of anti-fungal, like those already discussed, to finish off the job of bringing bad guys fully under control. Eventually, antifungals complete their work and no more die-off is experienced. The score on the candida questionnaire falls right down to its minimum level, reflecting the fact that the one-time sufferer now feels great!

For some people, die-off reaction is so severe that they seem unable to tolerate even the lowest level of antifungal supplements. The most probable explanation is an already toxic liver so, having ensured that they are drinking plenty of water and avoiding constipation by taking vitamin C to bowel tolerance levels *(see Chapter 3)*, I then suggest that they take a supplement containing the herb silymarin because this supports the liver and helps to reduce its toxic load. It is also helpful to drink dandelion root 'coffee' to help stimulate the production of bile, which carries toxins out of the liver. Sometimes it is necessary to take even further steps to detoxify the liver, and this was discussed in Chapter 4.

Another possible explanation for severe die-off reaction is that the immune system might be reacting 'allergically' to the presence of die-off toxins in the bloodstream. This situation often shows itself as depression or anxiety, which can be alleviated by taking supplements designed to reduce histamine levels, thus reducing the severity of die-off and enabling an easier climb up the antifungal ladder.

As we have seen, candidiasis is frequently not recognized or even acknowledged by medical practitioners, which often means that neither is it understood by family and friends. Die-off reaction, even when recognized and regulated by the sufferer, can lead to even more distress when friends and relations expect you to be getting better yet you are actually feeling worse and looking terrible! Loneliness and despair add to the physical and mental suffering created by the enemy within – and *Candida albicans* is one of the most vicious and relentless enemies there is.

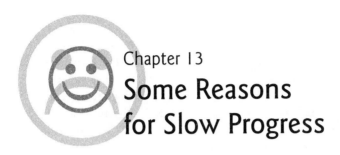

Chapter 13

Some Reasons
for Slow Progress

Occasionally, little or no progress seems to be made in the candida battle. When this is the case, there is always a reason which needs to be found. It might be that some other piece of unsuspected cargo is putting a load on the good ship *Immunity*, something like food intolerance or amalgam fillings in the teeth. Amalgam contains mercury which is a toxic metal. Its continual presence in the body requires the immune system to work extra hard. If nutritional steps to detoxify the body seem unable to cope with the situation, it is sometimes necessary to have amalgam replaced by less toxic fillings, but I have found that this is seldom a necessary step to take.

Perhaps little improvement is seen because the digestive system is not effectively breaking down food into nutrients which can be absorbed into the bloodstream, and so the immune system is not receiving the boost it requires. This can even mean that food supplement tablets pass straight through and out the other end, in which case they have obviously had no opportunity to do their work. If this problem is identified, it can be helped by taking digestive enzymes and possibly hydrochloric acid supplements for a while to boost the gastric juices.

It is an interesting phenomenon that either too little or too much hydrochloric acid in your stomach will cause exactly the same symptoms! So how do you tell what is happening? Quite simply, you eat some beetroot – cooked or raw, but not in vinegar. You then watch the colour of your urine, and if it appears red, this means that there was not enough hydrochloric acid in your stomach to break down the colouring in the beetroot. If your urine stays yellow, you may well have too much acid but the test is not sufficiently refined to say how much. All that you can be certain of is that, if your urine is red, your stomach is not making enough acid, in which case it needs some help. This is where hydrochloric acid supplements come in, but you also need to take steps to increase your acid production so that your stomach doesn't become dependent on the supplements. If you have vitamin B_6 and zinc in your supplement programme, this will help, as also will the amino acid L-Histidine, and drinking dandelion root 'coffee' 15 minutes before your meals will stimulate your gastric juices in readiness to digest the coming food.

It might be that there are environmental reasons for your hold-up. It is sad but true that your home could be making you ill. The house should be inspected for any damp or mouldy places, especially in the kitchen or bathroom but also round the frames of double-glazed windows, which need to be regularly wiped with an antifungal preparation. If you own some house-plants, the very air you breathe as you sit in your living-room will be full of air-borne spores rising from mould in the soil. You really need to find good foster-homes for your treasured plants and in their place, for Christmas and birthday presents, ask for some of the beautiful silk arrangements which are now available. It is amazing how often my clients do not take this caution seriously, because many of us are as sentimental about our plants as we are about our pets! The fact remains that it is likely to make an enormous difference to how ill or well you feel, because a candida-sensitive immune system will react to any of candida's yeasty relations, including mould.

Slow progress might be due to other environmental factors like domestic gas. This involves considerable detective work and maybe some unwanted financial outlay if you have to swap your gas cooker for an electric one and have your central heating changed as we once did after discovering that I was allergic to gas. All I can say is that the improvements it brought made it so worthwhile – and several years later we were able to have gas reinstalled, with a new boiler and two beautiful open gas fires!

The area in which you live might also play a part. Several people have told me that their illness began after they went to work in an oil refinery, or even went to live close to one, and chemical smells carried by a prevailing wind can sometimes lead to a definite worsening of symptoms. Even in the country, pesticide sprays put a tremendous load on the immune system, triggering asthma and other complications, and vast fields of rape seed in bloom ensure a difficult few weeks each year for a great many people. In autumn, rotting leaves can lead to a worsening of symptoms, and for me a holiday in beautiful Northumberland was once ruined by a visit to a musty castle!

There are many possible factors which might be delaying your progress, and it is important to consider each of the other possible pieces of cargo. For instance, constipation will increase all the symptoms of toxicity *(Chapter 4)* and diagnostic tests might be helpful to counteract the effects of stress *(Chapter 6)* or to uncover a hidden parasite *(Chapter 10)*. Read carefully through the chapters in which I have discussed the various pieces of cargo, and see if you can pinpoint some factor which as yet you might not have considered could be responsible for your slow progress to health.

Just occasionally, it has to be said, I discover that someone is not getting well simply because they are not being strict enough with the diet! Friends and relations persuade them to have a piece of Christmas cake, or some raspberries from the garden, or a glass of wine at a birthday dinner, and people are very good at saying things like, 'It can't *possibly* make any difference if you have just one little slice of cake!' Or, 'Everyone knows that fruit is *good* for you!' Or, 'Anyway, who says this diet is going to help you? Nothing has actually been *proved*, has it?' Or, 'You can always go back on the diet tomorrow, if you *really* think it's helping, but *I* think you've lost an *awful* lot of weight. It *can't* be good for you!' Bear in mind that people who have no self-discipline in their own eating habits often feel threatened by those who do!

It is absolutely essential to be totally motivated to sticking to the diet and to have the courage of your convictions in order to withstand such pressures from your nearest and dearest. Not to do so is a waste of your time and money and will certainly slow down the speed of your recovery. What's more, it will lead to another bout of die-off to live through – and you are the one who will have to endure it, not your sceptical mother-in-law! (Sorry, that is just said as a silly example. I don't mean to be rude to mothers-in-law – I am one myself three times over!)

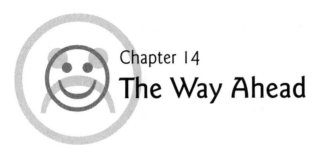

Chapter 14

The Way Ahead

There is no easy way to win the candida war. It takes courage, determination and perseverance – but it can be done. Even when you're nearly well, the effect of die-off toxins and unaccustomed exercise can make you feel that you are back at square one! *(Read about the lymphatic system in Chapter 4 – 'Toxicity and Pollution'.)* For more than 50 years, I fought an unidentified foe. In my own experience, the unmasking of the enemy was the initial breakthrough; the four-point plan brought victory, as you can read in my story in Chapter 16.

You will know that candida is under control when you are free of symptoms and when higher levels of antifungals produce no further die-off effects; it's as simple as that! It's a good idea to check your score on the candida questionnaire, to make sure it has reached its minimum level. In other words, all symptoms should have gone and only risk factors should remain to be counted in the score. The object then is to consolidate what you have just achieved in terms of establishing a new healthy balance of microbes in your intestines.

When the candida score sheet shows points for nothing more than risk factors (or almost). my plan of action is to experiment cautiously with relaxing the anti-candida diet just for a month in sensible ways, to see if this will cause a return of any previous symptoms. I suggest having a small amount of wholemeal yeasted bread, some crisp fruit (apple, pear), low-fat milk and some Edam or Gouda cheese, unless of course there is a known intolerance to dairy produce. It is sensible to continue taking anti-fungal supplements and acidophilus during this month to provide some 'insurance cover' in case the experiment turns out to be a little too soon and symptoms start to recur, in which case you need to return to the diet and increase antifungals again for a month or two longer and then try to relax the diet again.

However, if all goes well with the experiment, it is then safe to stop taking antifungals and acidophilus supplements but important to continue on a maintenance programme of vitamins and minerals to keep your immunity boosted. It is also necessary to return to the diet for a further year in order to consolidate the newly-established healthy balance of bacteria which will just have been achieved in your intestines. That's possibly the hardest part of all, because now you are well you probably have less motivation to stick to the diet any longer! However, you do have a little more leeway than previously to break the diet (sensibly!) if you are eating out or away from home on the odd occasion, but to do so every day or even every week at this stage would only serve to reactivate your resident candida before the good guys have had sufficient time to be strongly re-established.

You need to bear in mind that we can never completely rid our bodies of candida; we can only get rid of its overgrowths and make sure it's pushed back behind its 20-per-cent boundary-line. It would therefore be all too easy to reactivate it, especially at this early stage. Exercising self-control and patience for a further year is therefore so worthwhile because, at the end of the year, you will almost certainly find that you can transfer to a general healthy diet which includes wholemeal yeasted bread, fruit, cheese and perhaps even a little alcohol. As a nutritionist, I feel I have failed in my job if my clients have the slightest desire to return to sugar or junk foods, because the anti-candida regime is an excellent opportunity to learn how to enjoy eating all the delicious healthy foods which are available to us, and there is no point at all in returning to the very foods which encouraged your body to become ill in the first place.

I believe there is less chance of candida being reactivated in someone who has brought it under control and has also boosted his immune system to keep it that way than there is of someone experiencing its symptoms for the very first time. The difference is that once you have recovered from candidiasis you know how to live healthily to avoid a recurrence, whereas the person who has only just developed thrush or rectal irritation or other minor symptoms as yet has probably no idea that they are being caused by diet and other lifestyle factors! Anyway, who would knowingly *choose* to walk back into problems of sickness and despair once they have all been left behind?

Part ③

Feeling Great!

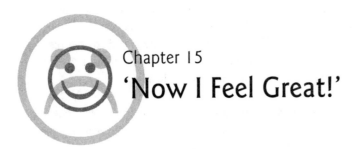

Chapter 15

'Now I Feel Great!'

For someone starting out on a nutritional regime, the road ahead can seem long and uncertain. Recommended changes in diet may be radical, affecting family and social life, and the cost of supplements reaching on into an indefinite future can be daunting, involving sacrifice and financial planning. Does the programme really have to be so strict and so demanding? In the end, is it really going to prove worthwhile?

If you are in the process of weighing up the possible pros and the undoubted cons, or if you simply need assurance that the nutritional advice you have decided to follow really is likely to bring some benefits, I suggest that you read the following accounts collected from several of my clients who, like you, had to adjust to a new way of eating, find money for supplements and consultations, frequently coping with die-off reaction from candida toxins and withdrawal symptoms from caffeine, and all the time wondering whether this really was the right thing to do and whether, in due course, they would actually reap some benefits!

I feel certain you will be encouraged – and who knows? *Your* name might well be one of those appearing in my next collection of testimonies!

Clive, a young man from Essex, had been diagnosed by his doctor as suffering from CFS/ME eight years previously, at the age of 19. He describes himself as going from happy and fit to depressive, ache-ridden and permanently tired. On doctor's advice he took anti-depressants and gave up sport. He says:

> These things didn't seem to make any difference and my life took a downhill turn. I stayed feeling dreadful for about three years during which time I had to give up a university course.
>
> For some unknown reason I gradually started to feel a little better but was still feeling worse rather than better for most of the time and needed large amounts of sleep. After a further five years of being very up and down I met Erica while servicing her computer! I started on the anti-candida diet which seemed very daunting at first but I was determined to get myself fully fit again.
>
> After the first three months I was starting to feel a bit better but not great. The die-off reaction of the antifungals was hard to handle because just as I was starting to feel better it would knock me down again. Fortunately with time these bouts got less frequent which made things easier.
>
> After a year on the diet I tried relaxing it for a month and had no side-effects so gave up the anti-fungal supplements. Going back on the diet for a further year, as Erica advises, has been no problem because I have found that I now prefer soya milk and soda bread to their 'yeasty' equivalents.
>
> I feel confident that I have kicked my ME/candida problems and am feeling fully fit for the first time in eight years. I can go to bed late and get up early without suffering the next day. Standing up and concentrating for long periods causes no problems and I can now say that I feel content with my life and don't worry much at all. It is great to feel so fit again after such a long time.

Elise, from Aberystwyth, had suffered from CFS/ME for eight years but also from other health problems all her life. She writes:

Two and a half years ago, after having my baby, I simply didn't get better. I'd eaten anything and everything during the pregnancy, and felt well at the time even though I know now that I had probably suffered seriously with candida since eight years ago, which was when ME set in. Out of desperation I contacted Erica and started immediately on the diet and vitamins and minerals she advised, adding caprylic acid (to kill yeast) and acidophilus supplements (to restore the friendly bacteria) a month later. Post-natal depression was severe for three months; belching, little appetite and fatigue due to die-off were severe, compounded by little sleep. Erica's supplements dealt with the post-natal depression also, so that within eight months I felt almost normal, but with not much energy. Although die-off was severe, at least I could control it by the dosage of antifungals and vitamin C intake. My lifelong problems started to disappear – after 'flaring-up' quite badly – such as cystitis and thrush, and by the first summer I was well, although still very tired.

Last summer I started to play badminton and was pleased with my level of fitness – the first time to have been fit in 15 years! It takes a long time, but perseverance pays off when you have help to know what you're doing.

Jill, from Swansea, had been medically diagnosed as having CFS/ME for more than two years. After she had followed my advice, I was thrilled to receive this letter:

Just a few lines to say many thanks for all your help and support since I started treatment for candida.

Before starting treatment I had been diagnosed with CFS/ME (of unknown cause – no virus was found) and had become so ill that I was bed-bound and house-bound for two years.

Before my illness I was an NHS Senior Physiotherapist and played a lot of sport, tennis and squash to a very high standard. I was amazed that the medical profession couldn't help me – all I was told was 'rest'!!

In my prayers I asked God to give me a sign if he was able to help me. Within days I saw your *Beat Candida Cookbook* advertised and after reading it I knew what was wrong with me! I started on a candida regime and slowly but surely I started to improve. I knew I was on the right track!!

During the times I felt discouraged along the way, you were always there with encouragement, help, support and enthusiasm. Your personal approach is invaluable to me and your other clients.

After six months of treatment, I have more energy, my head is clearing and my brain is working properly again! I can walk further and have started driving again short distances, also gentle swimming once a week. My quality of life has improved beyond recognition – it's wonderful!!

All my friends and family are amazed at my improvement. Every day I thank God.

Debbie, from Hampshire, had been diagnosed as suffering from Post Viral Fatigue Syndrome 19 months before she contacted me. Eleven months later, she wrote:

I feel like a new person! I am able to tackle mowing the lawn and other household tasks without collapsing in a heap for days afterwards. The improvement in my health and energy has been so remarkable that I don't regret embarking on this diet at all. A positive outlook, determination and an iron will are all that is needed!

When **Fiona**, from Essex, first contacted me, she had been diagnosed with Chronic Post Viral Fatigue Syndrome seven months previously, and was consulting a neurologist who had prescribed antidepressants. She had been too ill to continue her first year at university but, having first consulted me in January, she was fully fit and able to resume her studies in the Autumn term. She wrote her story for this book during the Christmas holidays, having successfully completed a full and happy term!

Having collapsed in a university lecture, I was told I would be ill for about two weeks. I waited with great frustration, only to find that three months later I still could not even walk. I had no memory or concentration. Despite feeling exhausted, I could never sleep until the early hours of the morning, and then would wake feeling as though I had run a marathon! I could not cope with light, noise or conversation. I had so many blood tests, the nurses joked that I might 'dry up'!

In pain and bed-ridden, I wondered what was happening to my body. Glandular fever was then diagnosed, but a few months later I was feeling even weaker. I struggled to get back to university but only managed two lectures in a whole term. I couldn't manage stairs and when I first went to the supermarket I just wanted to lie down in the middle of the aisle. My muscles still ached, especially when I used them!

Finally, I saw a neurologist who gave me a brain scan and told me I had a classic case of CFS/ME. He confirmed that my brain did actually exist but that it was working like a 'faulty computer programme'!

The university tried to encourage me to take a year out to recover. I eventually gave in and later discovered Erica's nutritional regime with the anti-candida diet. My headaches immediately disappeared; I had forgotten what life was like without them. From then on, my symptoms gradually left.

I am now relaxing the diet, having been on it for a year, and have completed a term back at university (including a game of hockey and an all-night Ball!). Friends are amazed at the speed of my recovery and it feels so good to have my health back. I have been challenged by the amount of sugar I was consuming. The diet has been the key to my recovery (along with the prayers of many friends). I have been really blessed and supported by Erica and her staff, and my eyes have been opened to the basic fact that what we eat will hugely affect our health and general well-being.

Mary, from London, was referred to me by her consultant neurologist who said that she fulfilled all the necessary criteria to meet a diagnosis of classic Chronic Fatigue Syndrome. She had been in good health until six years previously and, besides working as a nurse specialist in women's health, she had lived an active life in her family and church. Then in 1993 she was taken to hospital with a suspected pulmonary embolism, which transpired to be a viral infection. The chest pain continued and she became increasingly aware of debility and fatigue.

When she first came for a nutritional consultation, we identified several loads on her immune system as being poor glucose tolerance (low blood sugar), a low histamine status, extreme overweight, a rather poor heart profile including high blood pressure, stress, a fairly high pollution profile, and an overgrowth of candida. With her immune system labouring under all these loads, it really was not at all surprising that she had been unable to fight off a nasty virus when it attacked.

At the time she wrote the following words, Mary had not yet recovered 100 per cent full health, but the difference in just six months was enormous. Her candida 'score' had dropped from 176 in June to 64 in September and 17 in December. Another bonus was that her weight had dropped by almost 10 kg (22 pounds). With the light at the end of the tunnel drawing so close, it is almost certain that Mary will soon be fully well. Read her own words:

> Over the years, I have read many articles similar to my own story and hoped and prayed that one day it would happen to me! In 1993 I was admitted to hospital with chest pain and investigated for a pulmonary embolism. Instead, an Echovirus was diagnosed. The chest pain was extremely worrying because both my parents had died of sudden heart attacks, my mother when she was quite young. In my case, it seemed to be the beginning of Chronic Fatigue. After an initial four months' sick leave, I eventually returned to part-time

work but battled with tiredness, lack of energy, muscle fatigue, poor concentration and pain. Further blood tests and X-rays showed no abnormalities, which was disappointing because however dire the diagnosis I would have been relieved to know what was wrong. Unfortunately, at this stage, I was a very sceptical health-care worker as far as the diagnosis of Chronic Fatigue Syndrome was concerned!

During the coming months and years I pushed myself to work, collapsing in a heap at the end of the day and needing days or weeks of sick leave. As I was approaching the menopause, I took various prescriptions for hormone replacement, with very little improvement. Life for my husband and myself was affected badly by long, miserable days, having to go to bed early, not sleeping, then having vivid dreams, getting up late, resting and watching too much television. I didn't want to go out because noise or being with people seemed to exhaust me more, leaving me listless and very debilitated over the following days.

This picture continued until May 1999 when I commenced a structured programme as advised by my consultant neurologist, learning the very hard discipline of not pushing my body on good days and also of setting myself achievable tasks with periods of mental relaxation. In addition to this, in June 1999 I had a nutritional consultation, after which my diet completely changed. Initially it was hard because my eating habits had become quite poor due to my lack of energy and low self-esteem. However, the diet became part of my recovery and I began to realize how much better I was feeling. Admittedly the first few weeks were quite gruelling due to the 'die-off' effects of candida – even though I couldn't believe that my problem could possibly be candida as I had never experienced vaginal or oral thrush! I was amazed when I became aware of all the other candida-related symptoms and predisposing factors – burning watery eyes, dry mouth, bloating, cravings, constipation, nasal itching – the list is never-ending!

At first the combination of diet and supplements as well as the structured programme all seemed too much, but as my symptoms

143

declined so my enthusiasm for a fuller life developed. At that stage the problems lie in keeping to a sensible lifestyle without rushing into too much activity. I now work for short sessions without feeling exhausted at the end of the day, setting myself realistic goals and feeling pleased at the achievement. Friends and family quickly learned to accept 'my diet' and were greatly encouraged to see signs of the old 'me' returning.

It does all work despite the scepticism which unfortunately still abounds in some medical circles. There is still some way for me to go but I feel confident that with determination, the diet and nutritional support, the chronic fatigue becomes less chronic!

Paul, a 20-year-old computer enthusiast from Essex, was referred to me by the same consultant neurologist. He had been diagnosed as suffering from CFS for two-and-a-half years, and had suffered irritable bowel syndrome for the past 12 months. Part of his fatigue state was that he developed a recurrent sore throat and swollen glands whenever he experienced a relapse – which was quite regularly. He first came to see me in November 1998. The apparent loads on his immune system showed as stress, low blood sugar, caffeine (he drank 10 glasses of cola drink each day) and an overgrowth of candida. Read what Paul says in his own words:

I spent two years going up and down with my illness. Twice I managed to get nearly better, but then in a couple of days I would become as ill as I was to start with! Every time I started to get better, I would constantly worry about when I was going to get worse again. I couldn't plan to do anything in case I became too ill to do it. I had tried a number of things to get myself better; everything I tried helped to some extent but failed to lead to a full recovery. It was decided that I should see a nutritionist to see if improving my diet would help me get better.

I went to see Erica and she immediately told me why I wasn't getting better and decided on the best course of action. At this point I didn't really expect much – just a little boost like all the other treatments had given me, but after two weeks into the diet I became stable and felt comfortable with my situation. I then started to improve quite quickly, and found I could do more and more and not get tired. The strangest thing was that I wasn't worried about getting worse this time because everything just felt right. I kept on improving and improving and didn't get worse at all.

The diet was quite hard to get used to but I found that when the cupboards were full of food which I could eat (*well done, Mum!*) it became easy to stick to the diet. The best thing was that I could eat as much as I liked without having to worry about whether I should stop, like happens when you eat a big bar of chocolate!

It took a year for Paul's candida score to fall from 117 to just 20. Along the way he had a laboratory stool test from Great Smokies which showed that, besides an overgrowth of candida, his intestines were also infected with a type of staphylococcus bacteria. A suitable programme of antibacterial herbal supplements was introduced to fight it with obvious good results. We also discovered that he had an intolerance to dairy foods, so he has since avoided them. In less than a year from his first consultation, he returned to playing badminton and even went on a white-water rafting holiday in Turkey with no subsequent ill-effects! Even so, I had to warn him that with a score of 20 he was still in a fairly vulnerable position so he would really need to follow right through with his nutritional regime to ensure that his new-found health was stabilized. However, Paul showed such determination throughout and such a positive attitude to the anti-candida diet (even Christmas didn't daunt him!) that I have no doubt at all that he will both achieve and maintain a level of optimum health. He deserves it!

Derek, also from Essex, wrote his story and sent it to me. I'll let him speak for himself.

It was 4.00 a.m. one Friday morning in March 1996 and I awoke with a pain in the left side of my stomach. The pain would not go away despite frequent trips to the toilet and trying to lie still in bed. It had been another week of endless meetings, telephone calls in the middle of the night because of production concerns and regular visits to the pub to try and drown it all out. In 1996 I was a plant manager for a well-known car manufacturer that was going through a process of a shrinking work-force and financial budgets which meant for me an ever increasing workload with deadlines that had to be met. Nobody wanted to listen to my concerns and very often I would go to work in the morning and not return home till the following evening, having slept on the office floor. I had no family life; my life was my job and my job was my life, something I now deeply regret.

On that morning I dressed myself for work because I had to make an 'all important presentation'. But I was in pain, and after eight years of not taking a day off sick, I knew I needed help and so I called my wife to take me to the hospital. My wife dressed our two sons and we headed for the nearest hospital – only to find that it had no emergency department and we had to make a longer drive to the next hospital. My wife left me to take our sons to school and I sat alone, waiting to be seen by the doctors. The pain got so bad that I staggered to the nurses' office and said I was going to the toilet to be sick, which I never was. As I left the toilet two nurses took me into a consulting room where three independent readings showed that my blood pressure was 240/180! After 13 hours in hospital, the diagnosis was kidney stones and I was transferred to another hospital for the night. The following morning the hospital discharged me with an appointment to see a kidney specialist the following week.

May I ask you, as you read my story, do you have any faith or religious beliefs? Until this point I had worked in my local church helping with The Boys' Brigade. I had recently decided to become a Christian and I was to be baptised on Sunday, the day after I left hospital. To me it seemed that the start of my illness was God's way of telling me I was about to start a new life, and the next stage was baptism.

The kidney specialist informed me that I was all right and that I should return to my local doctor. My local doctor was very supportive and gave me reassurance at every point in my illness. I told her I felt better but I had a pain running down the right-hand side of my chest that was very severe. She immediately wrote a letter to the hospital and instructed me to return there that same afternoon. The hospital examined me and admitted me with a suspected heart attack and I spent the next eight days in a cardiac ward. I frequently had pains that started under the left-hand side of my rib cage and then ran up the middle of my chest and down my left arm to the tip of my middle finger. The pain now was so bad that I nearly passed out and the nurses gave me injections of morphine to relieve it. The hospital found no trace of a heart attack and discharged me after eight days with instructions to return to the kidney specialist.

The specialist could find nothing wrong and so he referred me to another specialist who came to the same conclusion but decided to refer me on to a consultant neurologist who, I was told, collected such patients as myself. My illness had dragged on for six months, but now I felt I was finally about to meet the person who could put my life back together again.

The first consultation with the neurologist lasted two hours and I remember two things from that first meeting. He asked me where I worked and upon hearing the answer he replied, 'I see loads of people from your company.' Then after the physical examination he asked if I liked my job. I replied, 'I love my job, I put it before anything else.' He replied that this was the reason why the company promoted me and why I was now with him! This comment immediately highlighted what I had done to my life and, more importantly, why I was ill. The consultant diagnosed Chronic Fatigue Syndrome and said it had probably been triggered by the fact that when I'd had flu five months before my illness began, I had not taken enough time off work to fully recover. I was prescribed a course of amitriptylene and appointments were made with a psychiatrist and an occupational therapist.

During the next 12 months I kept my various appointments, took the tablets and kept to my rest patterns. Life at home was hard for my two young sons because they did not understand what was wrong with Dad and why he could not go out with them. They also found it hard being quiet when Dad was having a rest period, but I think my wife found it the hardest. I was never around for the family when I was well and now that I was ill we could not function as family. I could not drive, walk far, answer the telephone or do any of the jobs around the house that needed doing.

Let me give you an insight into how I viewed other people and how I think they viewed me. If you have your leg or arm in plaster, have spots or sores on your body or are unconscious, then people understand that you are ill, but when they see a normal-looking human being who complains that he cannot do anything or is just too tired, they treat him with suspicion; certainly I experienced this. However, through the local church I made contact with a person who had been ill for a year longer than I had. We supported each other, tried different support groups and made contact with other sufferers in the area.

After approximately eight months of being ill, I went to a meeting with the doctor of the company where I worked and a person from the industrial relations department. My wife took me to the meeting and the first question I was asked by the industrial relations representative was, 'When do you think you will return to work?' At this my wife exploded and let out all her feelings about the situation. The doctor asked what were my work patterns and responsibilities and when I told him he turned to the industrial relations representative and said, 'Another one working crazy hours. When is it going to stop?' The reply was, 'When the rest of the management team have fallen over!'

We left this meeting in disbelief and my wife was shocked at how a large global company could treat its employees. Just before Christmas 1996 I went to see the Operations Manager who asked all the right questions and assured me that I would have a job to come back to. However, to keep the business running they would advertise my job for a replacement. My wife and I left the meeting with some faith restored in the company, only to have it dashed later when I found that my replacement was given an extra grade for the job.

I want to make the point that if qualified medical people state that you are suffering from Chronic Fatigue Syndrome, believe it. Don't worry about anybody else or what they think. If you are a carer or if you are responsible for a group of people working for you, I want you to try to understand what a sufferer of CFS experiences. Please don't try to tell them to have an early night's sleep or to snap out of it – because they cannot. If you feel you are a potential sufferer then look at your lifestyle and ask yourself if what you are doing is the best thing for your life and for others around you. I realize that once I was just another number, but now I have got the balance right between work and family life.

After approximately a year under the consultant neurologist, my health had improved to some extent but I believed I had certain food allergies. I had already stopped drinking alcohol and eating foods such as eggs, but I kept having annoying itchy rashes on my legs, which I would scratch until blood ran down them. At this point the neurologist sent me to see Erica and I can still remember the first appointment with her. After an hour I left having been told that I had to go on an anti-candida diet that would last in degrees for possibly two years. I could not have alcohol, fruit, sugar in any form, wheat products unless whole wheat, etc., and I had to take a whole range of food supplement tablets.

I have since met some sufferers who told me they could not keep to the diet or believe in it. I took the view that this was my 'medicine' and I was going to take it to get better. I have told Erica since that after our first meeting I did not believe food could affect someone in the way it did me. After three days on the diet I felt better, but when I passed water it was as green as grass. I learned later this was a sign of the high level of toxins in my body.

The more I progressed with the diet, the better I felt; the aching joints, the lack of motivation, the fuzzy heads all started to disappear. However, the best thing I did was to start taking regular exercise by walking every day and eventually I could walk three miles in 45 minutes. My weight when I was first ill was 232 pounds, but after two years on the diet I was not only feeling better but I weighed only 171 pounds. At the time of writing I have completed the two-year diet period and have been on my 'own' for some five months. I am still adhering to the basic diet with only the odd luxury now and again. Having gone through the diet and felt the benefits of it, I do not want to go backwards again.

I returned to work in February 1998, two years after my illness began, initially working just three hours per week. Since that time I have slowly increased my working time and it has taken me two more years to get back to working from 8.00 a.m. till 4.00 p.m., five days a week. I have certain responsibilities in my job, but I am in control of the hours I work. I am not slow in highlighting the situation if I think I cannot handle the workload and that I need help.

My family life is steadily improving and my two sons now want to do things with Dad, yet when I was first ill it took eight months before they would do things with Dad without Mum; Dad was always around, but never there. My future looks better than before and I have achieved many things that I would never even have thought about if I hadn't been forced to take time out from work. My family now comes first, and work is second in my life.

I hope you have taken comfort in reading my story and that you can identify with me in some of your own experiences and feelings. I started to doubt myself when I was ill and I learned about CFS the hard way by reading books and articles in magazines. It was only when I started attending support group meetings and read Erica's book, *M.E.: Sailing Free* (now enlarged and republished as the book which you hold in your hands!) that I realized I was not alone. What I was going through were real symptoms of a real illness. I try now to spend time with other sufferers and to encourage them by sharing my own experience and my achievements, and I am often asked for some points of advice, which I gladly share with you here:

1　If a qualified medical person tells you that you are suffering from Chronic Fatigue Syndrome, believe it and forget what everybody else tells you or thinks of you.

2　Ensure that you take the recommended rest patterns, tablets or exercise, because this is your 'medicine' to make you well.

3　If you think food is affecting you, no matter how strange it may seem, follow Erica's advice in this book and stick to it because again this is your 'medicine'.

4　Take regular daily exercise, no matter how little you start with. Do it, because if you do not, in my opinion the illness is likely to get worse.

5　Do not worry about getting back to work.

6　I found happiness and contentment in becoming a Christian. It gave me inner strength and courage. Perhaps you should consider this in your own life?

Finally, I wish you well in the fight against this illness. It's a fight you can win and I am proof of that. I wish you all God's blessings for a quick recovery.
Derek.

In compiling this little collection of encouraging experiences I have to give pride of place to the following, because it was written by a lady aged 91 who had suffered for several years with chronic fatigue, sinusitis, thrush and gout. **Elizabeth**, from Kent, wrote:

When I started work with you a year ago, I was on the eve of my 90th birthday. I count this as an advantage because it made me realize that I may not have very much time left for experimenting, and if relief from candidiasis can be achieved at this age, there is hope for a lot of other elderly people who may think they are too old to do anything about their own problems.

When I started I also had another advantage. I was already a convinced believer that optimum nutrition could and would act as a healing agent and I brought to your programme of treatment a feeling that if I kept to the regime for long enough and strictly enough, I should automatically get some relief, even if not a complete cure. Fortunately, I live alone and so can eat what and when I like, and this, again, is a great advantage for anyone starting such treatment.

For a number of years before beginning work with you, I had had very painful feet, which greatly hindered my walking. Also, I had become completely deaf, so much so that I could hear nothing at all. It felt like being in prison and out of the world. I also suffered from what is now known as Chronic Fatigue Syndrome. I was so tired all the time that I had to force myself to do even the simplest and most necessary things to keep going.

And now, after a year's faithful adherence to all your suggestions and recommendations, I feel a completely different person. The gout in my feet has completely gone; the catarrh in my ear, which had prevented me from hearing, is definitely clearing up, and I no longer wear a hearing aid as my hearing has improved so much. I am beginning to catch up with all the jobs I should have done long ago in my capacity as manager of a block of 32 flats. I also do all my own shopping and cooking and all the other things necessary to keep alive.

Is further comment needed?

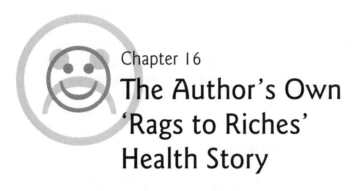

Chapter 16
The Author's Own 'Rags to Riches' Health Story

I hesitated at first to include my own story in this book because I was never diagnosed as having CFS or ME and I was therefore afraid it might seem inappropriate.

However, looking back over my life I now know that there were many times through the years when I might well have been given such a diagnosis, but this was 20, 30, even 40 years ago when the majority of doctors did not seem to be aware of a chronic fatigue syndrome – certainly none that I consulted in all those years.

Even without that diagnosis, I believe that there are many people who do have a diagnosis of CFS and who will be able to identify with much of my story, recognizing in their own lives the situations which I describe – and thereby finding hope that the outcome for them might be as good as it has been for me.

In addition, I believe there are probably thousands of sick people who, like me, have not been given a medically-recognized diagnosis and who are feeling that they've been left on a scrap heap. Maybe you are one of these, and by some 'chance' now find yourself reading this book. If so, I am certain that you will be able to identify with me in all the uncertainty as to what has gone wrong with your body, and I hope that this chapter in particular will help to show you at least a small speck of light at the end of your own long, dark tunnel.

As you read, you might be interested to look for the particular pieces of cargo which were weighing down my own good ship *Immunity* and causing it to sink, and see if any of these match up with your own!

Almost Sunk Without a Trace!

I have often said that I could not remember a day in my life when some part of my body did not draw attention to itself.

This isn't strictly true, for there were many 'sunny' days – playing in fields with childhood friends, Christmas in the cottage where I grew up, teenage fun, falling in love and an Easter wedding, then camping holidays and beach days with the children.

On so many levels, my life was really blessed. I was the only child of loving parents. Although the war was going on around and above us, it barely touched our lives in the country. I married a loving husband and we had three children who each brought great joy, as did eventually our three children-in-law and four (at the time of writing!) beautiful grandchildren.

Yet much of my life has been a nightmare, for interwoven through it all there was frequent sickness, affecting me not only physically but psychologically, too. There have in fact been very few days in my life when I have been totally free of some kind of illness, pain or anxiety.

Among my earliest memories are earache and thrush as a three-year-old. I can remember being sat in a bowl of 'something soothing' with an antiseptic smell, crying because I was so sore. That problem was never away for long. In addition, I had cold after cold and bilious attack after bilious attack. I was a bright enough child; I did well at school and enjoyed many friendships, yet the constant pattern of returning to school after illness became a nightmare to me, as time after time I had to rediscover my place in the world of children's relationships. In fact, I remember nothing but kindness and friendship from the village children, but I still dreaded the days when I would be well enough again to go back to school.

When I passed 'the scholarship' at 11 years old and had to travel daily by train to the Grammar School, my nervousness soon became school phobia. The reason for this, in addition to my constant ill-health and absences, was that I was terrified of the twice-weekly gymnastic lessons in which I might have to do a somersault, swing over the bar, or hang upside down on apparatus known as ribstalls. I would be physically sick with 'nerves' the night before a gym class. Eventually there were consultations between my mother and the headmistress, and special arrangements were made for me to be excused from those exercises, but nobody understood my fear – least of all me – or investigated the cause of it. It is only in recent years that I have realized that something was wrong with my balance, causing me to experience dreadful sensations in my head if I was in any position but upright and steady.

I was never without good friends, and have many happy memories of my teenage years. I was fit enough to enjoy long bicycle rides in the country, and to join a gang of friends for some memorable teenage hikes. But the heavy colds and bouts of influenza were still frequent and, in my early 20s, I began to suffer from sinusitis. Incredibly, this was not actually diagnosed for years, although I lived for much of the time with a 'spaced out' feeling in my head which I found hard to describe and no-one could really understand. At one stage the family doctor said I should have a holiday, which I did, but then I developed back pains and an upset tummy, so very little was achieved.

When I married Robin at the age of 23, it was still in the context of constant ill-health which continued to decline, happy though I was. The second year we were married, we lived in

London and I was working at the head office of a charity. One day in spring, I found it increasingly difficult to press the typewriter keys. Trying to ignore it, I went out at lunchtime but felt as though I was having to drag my legs along the pavement. Overcome with panic as to what was happening to me, I was helped back to the office where a taxi was called to take me home and a doctor sent for. Within an hour, I was at a hospital for nervous diseases, being examined all over by a medical consultant and a room full of students – but they could find nothing wrong with me!

Robin packed some things and drove me to my parents in the country, where my mother regularly massaged my limbs and took loving care of me. After a few months, the strange sensations of numbness and heaviness subsided – only to return in the spring of the following year – and the next, and the next, and the next! For 12 years it was a regular and dreaded occurrence. Obviously, the symptoms were due to allergy, and I was reacting to some type of pollen. The symptoms were systemic, affecting my nervous system and muscles, rather than 'straightforward' allergic reactions like hayfever or asthma, and this made it extremely difficult for a doctor to diagnose.

The general picture of my overall health was not improved by dreadful sickness in my three pregnancies, together with the nervous strain involved when two of our three babies became ill at three weeks old and needed operations for pyloric stenosis, a condition in which the stomach pumps up instead of down, leading to projectile vomiting and an increasingly starving baby. Added to this, just when our third baby became ill, I developed gallstones! Those who have experienced it will know that the pain of gallstones is unbelievably bad, and somehow I had to cope with it while at the same time trying to breast-feed a tiny baby who was fast losing weight because of projectile vomiting. Even after the relief and satisfactory outcome of the baby's operation, it didn't help to be told by a hospital specialist for six long months that my pain was nothing more than post-natal depression!

When baby Hannah was six months old and fully recovered from her operation, at last my gallstones were discovered and my gallbladder was removed, complete with stones. I went home to make a new beginning and start to enjoy my three young children. But two months later I was *really* ill! The 'spaced-out' feeling which I experienced quite often was now constant and severe. So were headaches, weak and aching muscles, stomach upsets, palpitations and anxiety. It began quite suddenly. Robin was travelling to Italy on a business trip that day, and I couldn't believe I was feeling so ill just because I was nervous that he was going away for a week.

The symptoms persisted even when he'd returned. Somehow I struggled on for a year, but for much of the time I was bed-bound. If I did manage to get to a shop at the end of our road, just a short walk away, I would have to spend the rest of the day on my bed, too weak to do anything else, my whole body shaking with palpitations. I needed to rely on friends and parents to help with the children, taking them to and from school and playgroup each day and even tidying their hair in the playground before they went in! I went away to spend two weeks with an aunt to see if a change and a break would help me to recover, and at first I still felt really ill – but by the second week things had definitely started to improve. I returned home feeling hopeful and encouraged but, within just a few hours, the symptoms had all returned. Could it all be psychological? We were beginning to think that it must be.

One Sunday, I was lying in bed feeling very much more dead than alive. Robin was trying to look after the children and also find ways of supporting me. I can remember feeling that I needed to fight to stay alive, and to do that I really needed to concentrate my mind on something engrossing – so we played game after game of 'Battleships' there on the bed, with pencils and pads of paper.

It was Sunday afternoon but Robin was so concerned about me that he had sent for the doctor. Eventually, an elderly locum arrived.

'How do you feel?' he asked.

'As though I'm dying,' was all I could say.

'Sounds like an allergy,' said the doctor, immediately.

He pulled up my nightdress and, using his thumbnail, drew lines across my tummy. As we watched, the thin scratch marks turned into wide, red weals, which stayed for a good 10 minutes.

'Just as I thought,' said the doctor. 'You can play noughts and crosses on an allergy patient!' And he wrote out a prescription for anti-histamine tablets.

Allergy again!

Once I became used to the drowsiness they caused, the tablets certainly helped. But what had caused the allergy? No-one seemed particularly bothered or able to find out. It was my mother who came up with an idea some time later and at first we simply laughed at her.

She suggested that I might be reacting to the new North Sea gas which had been installed in our area the previous year. (The talk at the time had been of 'conversion'; 'Have you been converted yet?'!)

My mother told us that her close friend had been suffering really badly from asthma ever since her gas supply had been changed, and she had no doubt as to the cause of her increased symptoms. Well, anything was worth a try! It was summer-time, so the only gas appliance in use was the cooker. I stayed upstairs in my bedroom for two whole weeks, with all doors firmly closed between me and the kitchen. Robin left me with supplies of food and drink each morning, so that I had no need to go into the kitchen. And by the end of the week, there was a marked improvement in how I felt! There was absolutely no doubt about it, so we quickly arranged to go 'all-electric' and, in spite of having little money to spare, we found a second-hand electric cooker and replaced a couple of gas room-heating appliances with second-hand electric nightstore heaters – incredibly heavy things which Robin had to transport manually, brick by brick.

Even all the gas pipes under the house were removed; we were determined to fight this problem in every possible way. I certainly was so much better for it – but sadly we soon made two more discoveries.

The first realization was that as soon as I went into other houses or buildings where there was gas, I would be ill for the next four or five days with all the symptoms of flu. It would happen whether I knew there was gas or not. Sometimes I would suddenly be ill and we would try to retrace my steps of the previous day – and invariably we would find a gas heater tucked behind a shop counter, or something similar.

The second realization was that I had become allergic to many other things besides gas, presumably because I had been exposed to the gas allergen for so long and it had worn down my immune system. In particular, the smell of paint would give me a blazing headache and set off many of my old symptoms. The worst problem was to find that I had become allergic to local anaesthetics, and the reaction was so severe that for the next 17 years I had all my dentistry without an anaesthetic, including three teeth crowned in one session! I remember the dentist afterwards saying, 'I don't know how you coped with that!', to which I replied, 'What choice did I have?'

In fact, it took a great deal of 'fight' to keep facing up to the constant problems, yet many people made it clear that they thought me a hypochondriac. A friend said to me one day, 'I won't ask you how you are; you're always ill.' She, and many others, had no idea of my constant struggle to find the physical and mental strength which were needed simply to keep myself going and face up to each new day and get through it.

By 1972, the wear and tear of it all had taken their toll of my body and my nerves. I experienced constant infections – sinusitis, 'flu', tummy bugs, kidney infections, cystitis, thrush, fibrositis – day in and day out. Added to this were the complications caused by the various allergies. Trying to bring up a family of three small children involved a daily battle with my body. I was exhausted, and exhaustion led to an anxiety state for which eventually my doctor prescribed some tranquillizers.

Allergies were a major problem, especially the spring-time syndrome which lasted every year from March till July, causing my arms and legs to feel weak and numb, and every possible muscle to ache. It was a time of year I dreaded.

One day in 1972, a friend called in and dropped a book in my lap. 'See what you think of that!', she said.

The book was called *Let's Get Well*, by Adelle Davis. I read it with amazement. Adelle wrote about all sorts of symptoms and conditions which I knew very well indeed from intimate personal experience, and she gave advice on how to tackle the problems with diet and vitamin and mineral supplements! Until then, I had honestly thought that you ate whatever you most enjoyed, and your body did its own thing. It had never before occurred to me that the two were closely connected!

The Tide Begins to Turn

Adelle Davis's book spoke a lot about which vitamins and minerals could be helpful for specific problems. I found it very interesting, and decided to try a few of her suggestions. She had written a lot about allergies, for which she recommended large doses of vitamin C and also Pantothenic acid (vitamin B_5) to help alleviate or even avoid the reactions. I tried it and it worked. In fact, it worked better than any of the antihistamine drugs I had ever been prescribed, and without the side-effects of drowsiness. I found that if I took these two supplements at breakfast, after half-an-hour I would start to feel very much better. Then towards midday the symptoms would start to return, but another dose at lunch-time pushed them away again. Four times daily I needed to take good levels of the two supplements providing vitamin C and Pantothenic acid, so the tablets went with me wherever I went, and made all the difference in the world to how I felt. It was truly amazing!

A whole new discovery had opened up to me – that nutrition affects the body! I suddenly realized that food is the fuel which makes our machinery work, just like petrol in a car. The fuel I had put into my body for the past 37 years had probably been about the lowest grade possible. I particularly liked sweet things!

What about coffee, which I drank several times each day? It didn't seem possible that coffee might be affecting my health in adverse ways; after all, it is part of our every-day culture. I decided to see what would happen if I gave it up for a while. The effect was dramatic and fairly immediate. Cystitis – that wretched complaint which had led me to sit in the doctor's waiting room more times than I cared to remember – completely disappeared!

In my discoveries about diet, I found something else which was very interesting. One of the health problems discussed by Adelle Davis was low blood sugar – hypoglycaemia. As I read through her case studies, I recognized myself. Very often, by late afternoon, I would collapse in a state of what I called 'my tea-time tizziness'. Quite suddenly, I would have to sit in a chair, absolutely still, unable even to turn my eyes sideways for fear of 'keeling over' and feeling far too weak to talk.

We had found how to get me through it. As soon as it happened, Robin would prepare a plate of food as quickly as he could and put it on my lap. I would eat it slowly, bite by bite, not moving my head or my eyes, until gradually the food would restore some strength to my body and, after a while, I would be able to talk to the children and cope with putting them to bed.

From Adelle Davis's description, I was certain that this was hypoglycaemia. Although she gave a fair amount of advice on how to overcome it, I felt I needed more information. It was going to be necessary, for one thing, to think through a radical change in diet, and also the vitamins and minerals which were evidently required would need a lot of working out. I needed more help – and it came!

One Sunday morning an unknown lady came and stood next to me in church. After the service, we started to chat. Veronica spoke with an American accent, though I discovered she was English by birth but had married an American and lived in the USA for many years. She had come over from Boston, Massachusetts, for the sad task of putting her elderly mother into a nursing home and selling up the family home and its contents. She was in England for a month and very lonely, living in a deserted house with gradually-lessening furniture. I invited her to come to us whenever she liked in the evenings, and we soon became good friends.

It just so happened that Veronica had suffered from hypoglycaemia but had been completely cured of it through following a special diet and taking a programme of vitamins and minerals recommended by doctors at an American clinic. She was able to help me with all that I needed to know and, when she returned to America, she sent me several books to help me even further. Among other things, I learned the importance of not eating sugar, and of having a snack containing protein every two hours. I took more vitamins as the books advised. And I began to feel *very* much better! No longer did my energy fade out at tea-time, so I could now enjoy the time of day when the children came in from school with their news. Increasingly, I was coming to understand the way in which food, together with vitamin and mineral supplements, could help my body to function more efficiently.

Slowly, surely, my health was being rebuilt. Yet often there were set-backs and for much of the time I still had sickness or pain. Even though allergies and blood sugar problems were now tremendously improved, it seemed as though there was still one heavy piece of cargo on board my *Immunity* ship which was keeping me pretty well submerged! What else did I need to discover?

In 1985 I heard about yeast infection. I was now regularly taking vitamins, which I ordered from a mail-order food supplement company. Occasionally, they would enclose fact sheets in the parcel and I would read about various health problems and the way they could be helped therapeutically through diet and vitamins and minerals. I was always interested to read these papers and one day I read one which was headed: 'The Spores That Attack You: When Your Immune System Can't Protect You!' The introduction said that a yeast which normally lives harmlessly in each one of us can also cause symptoms as diverse as runny nose, constipation, diarrhoea, bloated stomach, headaches, depression and infections of the vagina, kidneys and bladder, as well as many other problems. The yeast was called *Candida albicans*.

Conquering Candida!

My doctor said I could not possibly be suffering from yeast infection because, if I were, it would have cleared up with one week's antifungal treatment, which we had already tried for thrush.

However, the fact sheet said something very different – that it was difficult to bring candida under control but that it could be done with dedicated attention to diet (avoiding all yeasts and sugars), the inclusion of several vitamin and mineral supplements, and an anti-fungal drug called Nystatin which might be needed for several months. My doctor would not agree to prescribe the drug for me, so I decided I had to do what I could on my own and try to work out the diet. I thought it through and stuck to it faithfully but although I was convinced that I was on the right lines, the diet on its own made very little difference.

I had a friend called Moira, who also had a great many health problems. We believed that she, too, had 'yeast infection'. She decided to try the diet. In February 1987, Moira came to me and said, 'Guess what! My doctor has become interested in yeast infection and he wants to meet you!'

This was incredible! I had thought it would be quite impossible to find a doctor who would be interested in hearing what I had discovered, but now here was a doctor who wanted to meet *me*! I arranged to visit him and we spent an interesting hour, pooling our knowledge of *Candida albicans*, and he agreed to take me on as his patient. I transferred to his practice and he was happy to prescribe some Nystatin to try. He also gave me an even stricter diet to follow, which he had recently heard about.

I began to feel unbelievably depressed, to the point of being morbid. My sinuses and ears became extremely painful. I developed appalling pains in my mouth which seemed to come from the nerves in every single tooth and seared right through the roof of my mouth. There were days when I could not lift my face from the pillow because of the intensity of this throbbing pain. Things seemed to be getting worse instead of better.

After a while, I discovered that garlic oil had antifungal properties, and in desperation I tried applying it to my mouth in an attempt to relieve the pain – with very helpful results, initially. I started to 'paint' my mouth with garlic oil each night as I went to bed; fortunately, I have a very long-suffering husband! (I later discovered that garlic was not in fact helping the situation in the long term because of its ability to destroy friendly bacteria as well as yeast! These days I recommend an alcohol-free propolis tincture for this condition.)

This phase passed after a couple of months, and I continued to take Nystatin and to keep to the diet. Having come through the bad patch, things seemed to be pretty much as they were before.

At Christmas I became ill with some sort of virus, and I just couldn't seem to get over it. Week after week I sat by the fire, aching all over and totally lacking in energy. This had actually been the pattern many times before and I just waited for it to go away as it eventually always did. But this time it seemed to take longer. Some days I would think all day about the breakfast dishes waiting to be washed, but I didn't have the strength to drag myself to the sink to do it. On the rare occasions when I did manage it, I would stand and lean against the draining board, while the muscles in my back and legs just ached and ached and ached. For four months, it took more strength than I could muster to do that one simple task. I felt so guilty when Robin came home in the evenings and I still hadn't cleared the breakfast things.

By April 1988, I was still no better and I had come to realize that several of my friends, including Moira, were suffering from the same type of syndrome to a greater or lesser extent. About that time, I was lent a back copy of *Here's Health* magazine in which there was an appeal by students at the Institute for Optimum Nutrition in London for volunteers to take part in a research trial. They were looking into the effectiveness of a natural substance which was 'proving to be dramatically effective against the growing threat of *Candida albicans* infection'. The magazine was a few weeks out of date, but I quickly wrote off to see if I could volunteer for the trial. Eventually, I received a reply thanking me for my interest but stating that the researchers had found sufficient volunteers. Meanwhile, while I had been waiting to hear, I had done some detective work.

I asked at every health-food store and every pharmacy in my area if they had heard of this new substance or of the company (BioCare) which was marketing the product. None of them had, for it turned out to be a very new company. However, our local pharmacist kindly spent 30 minutes on the telephone till he tracked it down, and then I wrote to BioCare to ask for information.

They sent me some interesting literature which explained that the product was based on a fatty acid derived from coconuts. It had been known in the 1930s that certain fatty acids had antifungal properties and, in the 1950s, it was found that caprylic acid from coconuts had a fungicidal effect specifically against

Candida albicans. Caprylic acid products had been researched very thoroughly in America over the previous five years and, at the time of my discovery, they had been available in this country for only a few months. It was recommended that caprylic acid should be taken with other supplements known as probiotics, which would reintroduce friendly bacteria into the intestines.

I sent for both new supplements and carefully read the instructions. The recommendation was that caprylic acid should be taken at top dose straight away (12 capsules daily) because it was possible that at lower levels there might develop a resistant strain of yeast. I started to take the 12 capsules daily. For nearly three weeks, I noticed nothing – and then it hit me! Another enormous cloud of morbid depression descended upon me, interspersed with bouts of terrible anxiety. My ears became sore and thrush was severe. I ached in every muscle and I felt really ill all over. I didn't know what was happening, but I continued to take all the capsules.

Fortunately, later research showed that high levels of caprylic acid were not in fact necessary to avoid the development of resistant yeasts, so that it was therefore quite safe if taken at low levels. By this time I knew a great deal more about candida, and I was very glad to learn this information because it meant that no-one now would ever need to experience the horrendous symptoms which I had had to endure, caused as they were by high levels of caprylic acid destroying vast amounts of candida, which in turn had released enormous numbers of toxins into my body. This situation is commonly known as 'die-off reaction', but its official medical name is Herxheimer's reaction. I vowed that if ever I were to give advice on how to take caprylic acid, it would be to start with low levels and build it up gradually as die-off symptoms allowed, and this continues to be a vital part of the advice which I now give, as a qualified nutritionist, to my candida clients.

After a while, I started to feel better and people noticed a difference in me. They began to ask whether I could help them with their own health problems. I discovered Dr William Crook's candida questionnaire which was a good way of telling whether or not someone's health problems might be due to yeast infection and, if so, to what extent. If they had a high score, I told them about the anti-candida diet I was following and the various supplements that I took. Several people launched themselves into the same type of programme.

The real breakthrough in my health came towards the end of June, about three months after I had started to take caprylic acid and probiotic tablets. Hannah, by then at university in Cardiff, was due home for the long summer holidays. As it was the end of the academic year, she needed to bring a lot of her belongings home with her. Somebody had to collect her by car and, as Robin was away at the time on a three-month Christian training course in Sussex, it had to be *me*! I had never in my life driven more than a few miles at a time – 20 at the most – because I would so quickly become fatigued and, in any case, my health was so unreliable that it was likely to let me down at any moment! Now I was considering driving over 200 miles, alone, from Essex to Cardiff, and then back again with Hannah – and I was looking forward to it. Something was very different!

I stayed two nights in Wales and drove with Hannah for a day's walking in the Brecon Beacons, and the next day we went to a beach on the Gower Peninsula, and on the way home to Essex we went to visit Robin in Sussex. In four days I had driven over 900 miles. My health had been fine and I had enjoyed every minute. I even coped with having to call out the Automobile Association when my car broke down on the motorway!

Although at that stage I found that I still had recurring thrush and a less-than-perfect immune system, for the most part I now felt well and had more stamina than I could ever remember. There is all the difference in the world between being ill and being well apart from a few odd symptoms! I felt sure that before too long the remaining problems would catch up with the improvements already made.

Nutrition Training

My new-found health was clearly visible and made an impact on many people, including my doctor. I received more and more telephone calls from people asking if I could help them, as word seemed to spread like wildfire that I had found an answer to my chronic health problems. Each time I was asked for advice, I was very aware of my dreadfully inadequate knowledge but I also became increasingly conscious of the enormous number of people who were having to put up with chronic ill-health and desperately seeking for answers which the medical profession seemed unable to provide.

One day I came across a notice in *Here's Health* magazine publicizing a two-year Diploma Course at the Institute for Optimum Nutrition in London, to provide training for would-be Nutrition Consultants. Was this perhaps what I should do? Would a grandmother be accepted as a student? The course was pretty expensive; could we afford it?

These and other questions kept buzzing round my head, but the idea of training to become a Nutrition Consultant just wouldn't go away. I telephoned the Institute to make some enquiries and was invited to one of their Open Days for an interview. It so happened that I could manage none of the dates they offered, because of family holidays or other engagements, and I expressed disappointment. However, after a few more questions, I was offered an interview by telephone, which seemed second-best but at least would enable me to follow through with the possibility of training and to find out more about it.

The interview went well and I was offered a place for the Autumn term. What *had* I done? How much study would I have to do, and to what standard? I had left school at 17 with some good exam results and then had taken a year's secretarial course at the City of London College, where I had gained more certificates, but that had been the extent of my academic career, and it had ended 35 years ago! With this humble level of educational achievement, which was below the normal requirements for the I.O.N. course, I was given to understand that the reason I had been accepted was because of my obvious knowledge and enthusiasm for the subject and the fact that I was already involved in giving basic nutritional advice to many people who were requesting it. The interviewer obviously felt that I was the right sort of material to become a Nutrition Consultant!

One of the requirements of the Institute was that students without a scientific background should first of all enrol for a science foundation course, lasting just a few months, to study the basics of biochemistry. I had no science achievements among my age-old school certificates, so I certainly needed to do this basic study. I went to London for the first weekend of the course, and came home completely blinded by science! It was like having to learn a whole new language and wrap my mind around some totally new and bewildering concepts. Would I be struggling like this through two long years? I was never more grateful for my husband, because he had a university degree in Natural Sciences from Cambridge, and for the past 13 years had been teaching science to high school students!

I needed to ask him some pretty basic questions, and he patiently helped me to understand. Towards the end of the introductory science course, we spent a week in our caravan in Wales and devoted part of every day to going through my heavy textbooks together. Robin says that at the start of the course my understanding of science was that of a first-year high school student. By the end of the course, I had reached first-year university level! It seemed that my brain had received a kick-start and was getting nicely into gear.

I had enrolled at I.O.N. as a 'satellite' student, which meant that the regular lectures were sent to me on audiotapes. I studied at home and submitted my written work by post, but I also had to attend the Institute for several weekends in each year for workshops or seminars with my group tutor, Patrick Holford, who had founded the Institute a few years before.

Having completed the foundation course, I looked at the syllabus of work ahead and felt completely overwhelmed. It covered the physiology of all the major body systems and the part played by specific nutrients in the efficient functioning of each one. In addition, there would be lectures on such things as helping the body to deal with the effects of pollution, the politics of the food industry, when to refer clients to their doctor, etc., etc. It also covered workshops on giving public presentations and preparing press releases and many other aspects of working as a Nutrition Consultant. We would of course be learning how to calculate nutritional requirements from an analysis of symptoms in a client's questionnaire, and how to formulate an appropriate tailor-made supplement programme. It was all going to be extremely interesting, but there was so much of it! At the end of each of the two years there would be an examination, the final one covering the whole two years' work, and in the second year it would be necessary to submit case studies of 38 clients, some with three-month and six-month follow-ups. Most worrying of all, in the second year we would have to plan, carry out and write up a research project!

The reading list was heavy, literally! We bought some bookshelves and a desk from a second-hand furniture shop and these were put into our smallest bedroom which was fast becoming a combined study and office because, besides studying, I was also getting busier in another direction. People were becoming well through following my elementary nutritional advice, even though as yet I knew so little, but word of mouth was spreading and we were beginning to get telephone calls from people where we couldn't even trace the contact! All I could tell them was that I was not yet a nutritionist so I was not qualified to give advice and I was not insured to practise – but that I had been able to help myself with a certain diet and specific food supplements and it was entirely up to them if they wanted to try the same things. More often than not, they did, and I needed a card index system to keep note of all these contacts.

At one stage our local paper carried a disparaging article about CFS/ME entitled, 'Yuppie Flu', and I was incensed enough to write a letter explaining what I had so far discovered about the illness. As a result, I was interviewed and an article was printed which triggered so much interest that two weeks later a second article was run and this time, without my knowledge, it gave my telephone number at the end.

In the next two days I received 72 calls from sufferers of CFS who were desperate for help. I told them as much as I could, and agreed to obtain antifungal supplements for them if they asked me to. The telephone never stopped ringing, and we had to leave it off the hook at mealtimes in order to have some peace, so the next things needed were an answerphone and a second telephone line to make it possible for our family to get through to us!

The growing numbers of calls and letters to and from distant people were taking up a lot of time, so that my studying frequently had to be done very late at night, and yet my stamina didn't give out. I still was experiencing a few minor symptoms, but basically I was *well*! I had never before experienced such ongoing good-health, yet just a few months earlier it had seemed quite impossible that I would ever again have energy to wash the dishes!

Homework marks began to come in, and they were encouraging. Perhaps I could do it, after all! I found I enjoyed studying. For my research project, I chose to set up a trial on a nutritional approach to eating disorders. I knew how anorexia and bulimia could shatter the lives of sufferers and their families, but I had also discovered that nutrition, in particular the use of broad-spectrum amino acid supplements, could make a tremendous difference. I was glad to have an opportunity to test this out and to strengthen my growing conviction that the majority of eating disorders have a *physical* cause at their root, and are not just due to a psychological cause as is generally accepted. I co-opted help from the local press to find volunteers, and eventually had some very encouraging results. One lady, who had suffered with bulimia for 30 years and also with severe multiple joint pain, was completely free of both conditions after just 10 weeks of nutritional guidance!

During those two years of study and increasing requests for help, I coped with several family responsibilities, as well. Granddaughter Grace was born, and I spent 10 days helping out in Emma's household. My mother was twice in hospital, severely ill with pancreatitis, and I managed to visit her daily and also look after her flat. Hannah needed someone to type her project report for her degree in ophthalmic optics so I did that for her in the Easter break. Somehow everything got done, and my health and strength continued to hold out.

The two years flew by, culminating in October 1990 with my graduation. Out of 46 students completing the course, I had come first – a clear indication that hard work and enthusiasm pay off! Meanwhile, the contacts from people continued to snowball, and we decided we just had to 'go for it'. Robin handed in his notice at school so that he could stop teaching and join me in the work in order to take over the administration of the practice. My friend Moira helped part-time in the office and was a tremendous support throughout. Having a four-bedroomed house and with our children all flown from the nest, we were able to use one bedroom as a consulting room and one as an office. We had to think of systems to cope with the workload, and our son Toby, now living with his family near Leeds, designed some helpful programs for use on a small computer –

our first step into the world of hi-tech business! Before long, a team of assistants began to grow, until at the time of writing we have a team of seven in addition to two other qualified nutritionists who now take some of my workload! Last year we set up a company called Nutritionhelp Ltd., and under this umbrella we are helped by several Associate Nutritionists living all around the UK, and this enables us to cope with an ever-increasing demand for nutritional advice from postal clients all over the world, while others visit my practice for a personal consultation.

Three years after qualifying, I undertook an additional year of study because the Nutrition Consultant's course had been extended from two to three years and I very much wanted to upgrade my qualification to be in line with the new standards. For my required dissertation during that year, I researched and discussed the controversy surrounding candidiasis and a nutritional approach to its management. By the time I had looked at available research papers and medical text books, and was questioned on the contents of my dissertation for the final viva examination, I felt that I knew candida even more intimately than before!

I was invited to lecture at the Institute for Optimum Nutrition on what had become my two 'pet subjects', candidiasis and CFS/ME; later, I went on to lecture in Practice Management and Client/Consultant Relationships. What a long way I had come in a short space of time! For two years I also tutored third-year students, but eventually I found that this was just a little *too* much to fit in with my very demanding workload, so I sadly resigned as tutor – partly, I must admit, as a minor concession to the fact that I had reached the age of 60!

In 1990, Gill Jacobs (now on the Council of Management of *Action for M.E. and Chronic Fatigue*) contacted me and asked if she could include my story in a book she was writing, to be entitled, *Candida albicans: Yeast and Your Health*. This was eventually published and led to a large number of enquiries, many from people who said, 'Your story has such a happy ending!'. Gill has twice updated her book but my story has appeared in each edition and I still receive requests for help from people who have read it.

In 1991, I wrote and self-published the *Beat Candida Cookbook*, initially just to help my clients but it soon became popular with other sufferers and practitioners also. Without having any means for distributing it to booksellers, it sold over 11,000 copies in its original home-spun format. In 1999, I rewrote and revamped it for re-publication by Thorsons so that it now reaches readers worldwide. Very early on, I managed to develop a technique for undertaking consultations by post, which means that I have been able to advise clients anywhere in the world, and this side of the work continues to expand with the help of my Associate Nutritionists. I even responded to an invitation from clients in Dubai to give some presentations there, an experience I could never have dreamed of! I have found that I have a real love for giving talks and lectures and accept as many invitations as I can. A recent departure is an invitation from the College of Naturopathic and Complementary Medicine to lecture to their students in London, Dublin and Belfast and I have also enjoyed several opportunities to be interviewed on London's 'Premier Radio'. As a Christian, I am invited to speak at a growing number of conferences, and sometimes Robin and I will share the platform if we are giving a whole-day seminar.

I also love writing, and have enjoyed the challenge of having three books published within 18 months and of writing a regular column for a magazine called *Wholeness*. Having spent so much of my life in bed or slumped in a chair, at 65 it is great to wake up and wonder 'What's the next exciting thing that's going to happen today?'

A book called, *The Practical Guide to Candida* by Jane McWhirter, first published in 1995, makes gracious comments about my work and about the *Beat Candida Cookbook*. A classic on the subject of candida is Leon Chaitow's, *Candida albicans: Could Yeast Be Your Problem?* Published as long ago as 1985, it was the first book on the British scene, building on previous American publications by Dr Orion Truss and later by Dr William Crook. It is good that the role of candida in chronic health problems is being placed increasingly on the map by writers who have a good understanding of the problem, though often you will find that advice differs slightly from author to author.

Occasionally, I receive encouraging feed-back from doctors. I have been involved with various conditions, including heart disease and schizophrenia, where there has been approving comment from the hospital specialist involved. For some time I worked closely with the National ME Centre in England, receiving many referrals for nutritional advice from the Consultant Neurologist there. I think my most prized comment was made by a doctor in Yorkshire who read the report I had prepared for his patient and said, 'This lassie knows what she's on about!'.

Nutritionists do not claim to have a cure for any illness, but we do claim to be able to help each person achieve a status of optimum nutrition where many health problems simply cannot exist. It is obvious, if you think about it, that both the body and the mind will work better if they are optimally nourished – which means supplying necessary levels of vitamins and minerals to repair damaged cells and correct biochemical imbalances.

More about Candida

When I first learned about *Candida albicans*, it was like finding a missing piece of jigsaw puzzle. It explained so many things that had been happening in my body.

For one thing, I discovered that this yeast seems to love to inhabit old injury sites such as the knees or back. At the age of 18, I had fallen down some concrete steps onto a station platform, causing excruciating pain and severe bruising. After five years of suffering from repeated episodes of an apparent 'slipped disc', I was eventually shown by an osteopath that one of my vertebrae had been knocked sideways. (Several hospital specialists had failed to spot this on the X-rays.) Although osteopathic treatment and exercise helped me to recover from the initial injury, it left me with an extremely weak and painful spine for many years but since candida has been under control in my body, I have virtually forgotten the problems with my back that recurred with depressing regularity for more than 30 years.

I came to understand why I had to abandon any attempts to make bread or wine, even though at one time we bought ourselves jars and corks and all the paraphernalia of a wine-making kit! The incredibly severe headaches which flattened me on each occasion meant it was quite impossible to continue with our wine-making dream. Now I understood that the overgrowth of yeast in my body had made my immune system hypersensitive to yeast in the environment – which was therefore best avoided.

It was actually quite encouraging to discover that there were in fact other people like me who had become allergic to local anaesthetics, in spite of the fact that one dental specialist told me this was simply not possible and that quite obviously I was the type of woman who would faint if I saw a needle! (I couldn't help wondering how *he* would cope if he had to have three teeth drilled and crowns fitted all in one session without the luxury of a local anaesthetic, as I once did. Give me a needle any day!)

While on the subject of teeth, at one stage my dentist advised me to have some old crowns removed and replaced. They had moved very slightly over the years, leaving a small gap below the gum line. I felt that candida might be hiding inside these crowns, because if ever I had a flare-up of symptoms, it started in that area of my mouth. As the old crowns were removed, I could *smell* the infection inside them. Whether this was fungal or bacterial, I don't know, but either way it meant that my immune system had fewer battles on its hands once my nice new teeth were firmly fitted in place!

Other people also reported severe reactions to medicines and drugs prescribed by the doctor, just as I had so often experienced. This too was encouraging – for me, if not for them! So often, antibiotics had created a horrendous sense of panic, and I remember nights when I walked round and round the bedroom in what seemed like an attempt to keep my sanity, yet the panic subsided as soon as the effects of the antibiotic wore off. On one occasion, the doctor prescribed some pills for a tummy upset. In a very short space of time I felt as though the room had gone dark, I could hardly see and I could barely move. I crawled on all fours to the telephone and gaspingly told my doctor what was happening. He seemed not at all perturbed and told me to eat some bread and Marmite – for what reason I was never clear! After some hours, the effects began to go; it was as though a light had been switched on in the room and I could see again. I was left feeling weak and grey, and vowed never to touch that particular drug again!

When I first learned about candida and became convinced that this was the basic cause of all my problems, it came as a great relief. For years I had felt that I was disintegrating in all directions; now I knew there was just one major problem for which I needed to find the answer.

I realized, too, that although the vitamins I had been taking for several years had played a significant part in my recovery, it would have been much more effective had I known exactly what to take and how much of it! I knew that this boosting of the immune system had to be a vital part of any strategy which attempted to overthrow candida.

So, both from my own experience and then from the training I received, I found I had put together a four-point plan to recommend to other candida sufferers. Increasingly, as I gave this advice, I saw an astonishing number of people becoming well.

The first time I tried to help someone who had been medically diagnosed with CFS, I realized that candida was playing at least some part in his illness. This was a man in his early 40s who had been unable to work for over two years and who could only just walk from his car with the aid of a stick. After five months on a nutritional anti-candida regime, he was able to return to work!

He was the first of many, but I found that for some it takes a considerably longer time. These folk require even greater measures of patience, perseverance and determination. I have known a very few people who have become well in just three months; others have taken over a year, especially if they have been house-bound or bed-bound for a long time beforehand. The experience of most people with candidiasis falls somewhere in between, taking them perhaps six to nine months or even up to a year to feel completely well. It is impossible to say in advance how long it will take, because everyone is so completely different. People who have never taken the Pill or used steroids and who do not smoke will usually recover more quickly than those whose history is full of immune-suppressing medication or alcohol or drugs or those who are determined to keep on smoking!

Yeast infection is a wretched complaint from beginning to end, for even the process of getting rid of it is seldom a joy-ride. How good to know that we *can* break free of its hold on our lives!

Sailing Free!

The understanding I have gathered regarding a nutritional approach to overcoming health problems came about first of all as the result of my own improvements in health, followed by three years of training in optimum nutrition and then increasing experience as I saw an enormous number of people respond to nutritional advice. For me, it has been like living in an adventure story which has become more and more exciting as I have turned each page! How did it all come about? There is only one answer I can give; through faith.

Alongside my story of physical discoveries, there also ran an exciting thread of growing awareness in my spiritual life. Although I had been a Christian for many years, I still had a great deal to learn about God's love and power and his desire to bless me with health and in other ways, but that's another story which you can read in another book entitled *Doughnuts and Temples*. However, in Part Five I am including a discussion on nutrition from a Christian perspective. The first four parts stand complete in themselves as a nutritional approach to CFS and I do not wish to persuade you to read Part Five unless you have a specific interest in considering my thoughts on another aspect of healing and wholeness.

So, if you end your reading here, I hope you have been inspired by my own 'rags to riches' story (in terms of health!) and that you now feel it might conceivably be possible for you to look forward to health in the future. Whether or not my own years of illness could or should have been diagnosed and labelled as CFS/ME, I am certain that many who read this book will have identified with at least some of the suffering and symptoms which I experienced, and will have recognized in themselves the pieces of cargo which were placing a load on my particular *Immunity ship* – allergy, pollution, low blood sugar, stress, nutritional deficiencies, toxicity and candida, at the very least!

With such pieces of cargo – and possibly others – able to be identified in your own life and then off-loaded, I pray that your cargo ship, too, will be able to 'sail free' as mine has done!

Part **4**

'Let food be your medicine…'

(Hippocrates)

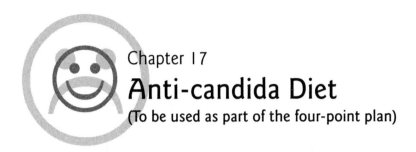

Chapter 17

Anti-candida Diet
(To be used as part of the four-point plan)

Foods to Avoid: ☹

☹ SUGAR, in all its forms, and food containing sugar. This
includes brown or white sugar, demerara, molasses, syrup,
honey, malt, chocolate and all other forms of confectionery,
icing, marzipan, ice-cream, desserts and puddings, cakes and
biscuits, soft drinks including squash and all canned drinks,
tinned fruit in syrup, etc. Check all tins and packets for
hidden sugar – even some frozen and tinned vegetables!
Types of sugar include fructose, lactose, maltose, sucrose and
dextrose.

☹ YEAST – all food containing it or derived from it. This includes
bread, food coated in breadcrumbs, Marmite, Vecon, Bovril,
Bisto, Oxo, etc., citric acid, monosodium glutamate, vitamin
tablets unless the label specifically states 'yeast-free', pizza
bases and most makes of pitta bread. Beware of commercial
wrapped bread which claims to have no added yeast if it has
been made with sourdough or sprouted grains because these
products have been fermented and contain their own
naturally-produced yeasts.

⊗ REFINED GRAINS – white flour, granary flour (which is white flour with malt and added whole grains), white rice, white pasta, cornflour, custard powder, cornflakes and cereals (unless 'whole grain' or 'wholemeal' is stated).

⊗ MALTED PRODUCTS – some cereals (e.g. Weetabix), some crispbreads, granary bread, malted drinks like Ovaltine, Horlicks and Caro.

⊗ ANYTHING FERMENTED – vinegar and foods containing it (ketchups, pickles, salad cream, baked beans), also soya sauce, sourdough bread, ginger beer, cider, beer and wine. In fact all alcohol, including spirits, acts as a stimulant which triggers the release of your sugar stores.

⊗ COW'S MILK and most milk products, including cream and most cheeses. *(See following notes about yoghurt, cottage cheese and butter.)*

⊗ FRESH FRUIT, raw, stewed, made into jam or juice. (Pure fruit juice is virtually 'straight' fructose and often also very high in mould!) Freshly-squeezed lemon juice is allowed in salad dressing, mineral water, etc.

⊗ DRIED FRUIT, including prunes and the fruit in muesli. N.B. Figs or dates are used to sweeten some health drinks (e.g. Caro, Bambu, Nocaff).

⊗ NUTS, unless freshly cracked, because of mould. Avoid peanuts completely, even in their shells (monkey nuts) because they are very high in mould. Avoid peanut butter for this reason.

⊗ SMOKED OR CURED fish and meat, including ham, bacon (even unsmoked is still cured) and smoked salmon, smoked mackerel, smoked haddock.

⊗ MUSHROOMS, which are a fungus. (So are truffles!)

⊗ TEA AND COFFEE – even decaffeinated, because they still contain other stimulants. Also avoid HOT CHOCOLATE.

⊗ COLA DRINKS AND LUCOZADE; they both contain caffeine, as do BEECHAM'S POWDERS and SOME PAINKILLERS (e.g. Anadin, Phensic, Panadol Extra).

⊗ ARTIFICIAL SWEETENERS, which have been found to feed candida just as effectively as sugar, and in any case keep your sweet tooth alive.

⊗ PRESERVATIVES, including citric acid, which are frequently derived from yeasts and in any case introduce chemicals to the body. (N.B. Sausages, even without preservatives, are high in animal fat and refined cereal.)

⊗ HOT SPICES AND CURRIES because they destroy friendly bacteria in the intestines.

Worried? You needn't be! Coming next are lots of enjoyable alternatives. And in Chapters 18 and 19 you will find menus and recipes to help you see how interesting and enjoyable the anti-candida diet can be!

Please note: Some medications encourage the growth of yeast, especially antibiotics and steroids (including creams and inhalers, the contraceptive pill and HRT) and NSAIDs (non-steroidal anti-inflammatory drugs). Also, rid your home of mould or damp – regularly clean around double-glazed windows – and get rid of all your houseplants; mould from the soil becomes airborne and could be keeping you ill.

Foods to enjoy: ☺

☺ YEAST-FREE SODA BREAD made with wholewheat flour or other grains. Some bakers will make a batch for your freezer.

☺ RICE CAKES (may be lightly toasted), OAT CAKES (malt-free), ORIGINAL or SESAME RYVITA, WHOLEWHEAT CRISPBREADS (read labels carefully).

☺ PASTRY made with wholemeal flour, oatmeal and sunflower or olive oil, in proportions of 3:2:2. Make very moist with plenty of water and dust well with flour before rolling.

☺ SOYA MILK or RICE DREAM as milk alternatives. (Different makes of soya milk have very different flavours.)

☺ BUTTER for spreading or cooking; otherwise for cooking use extra virgin olive oil.

☺ UNHYDROGENATED MARGARINE. Read the labels to make sure you pick the right ones. Avoid those with citric acid.

☺ COLD-PRESSED OILS: sunflower, safflower, linseed, as salad dressing mixed with lemon juice, and with an egg for mayonnaise.

☺ NATURAL YOGHURT (low-fat, unflavoured): try it for dessert or breakfast with lecithin granules or a mixture of seeds, or with a cereal like whole puffed rice. Spread it on top of wholewheat lasagne dishes before baking, or flavour with mint as a dip.

☺ COTTAGE CHEESE, as a spread or a filler for your jacket potato or with salad.

☺ BREAKFASTS: home-made muesli with oatflakes and other whole grains mixed with seeds, soaked in water and eaten with soya milk, rice milk or natural yoghurt; Shredded Wheat with soya milk or rice milk; puffed oats, puffed wheat or puffed rice or Kashi (mixed whole grains) with soya milk or rice milk; porridge made with water or soya milk, sprinkled with cinnamon or nutmeg and eaten with yoghurt; egg (boiled, poached or scrambled) eaten with wholewheat soda bread or toast and butter; rice cakes with cottage cheese and sliced tomato; slices of tinned pease pudding with tomato, grilled or heated in the microwave – and many more besides!

☺ MAIN MEALS: try to find a butcher selling free-range chickens and 'organic' lean meat to avoid hormones and antibiotics (lamb and rabbit are less likely to be affected), but don't forget that red meat has inflammatory properties. Enjoy any type of fish, but oily fish is particularly beneficial (herrings, sardines, mackerel, pilchards, salmon, tuna and trout). Combine a grain with a pulse for a complete vegetarian protein, e.g. bean and vegetable pie or crumble, rice or bulgar with chickpeas in a tomato or soya milk and herb sauce, whole wheat spaghetti or brown rice pasta twirls with brown lentils, tomatoes and onions.

☺ FRESH VEGETABLES of all types, steamed. Aim to have a plateful of SALAD, including TOMATOES, every day.

☺ AVOCADOS are good filled with cottage cheese and humus, or yoghurt with tomato purée, and topped with slices of cucumber.

☺ LEMONS; apart from avocados, the only fruit allowed. If adding a slice to your drinks, first scrub the peel well to remove traces of mould. Use lemon juice for salad dressing, for a yoghurt sauce with casseroled chicken and for squeezing over your fish.

☺ SEEDS AND FRESHLY CRACKED NUTS (not peanuts) make nutritious snacks. Choose seeds from sunflower, pumpkin, flax and sesame. Keep in the fridge. N.B. Shelled nuts have unseen mould.

☺ HERBS of all kinds, fresh or dried, add interesting variations in flavour to your meals.

☺ MILD SPICES also add interest (cinnamon, coriander, cumin, turmeric, etc.) but avoid the hot ones, especially chilli.

☺ HOT DRINKS: Barleycup and any type of herb tea or fruit tea provided it has no added citric acid or malt or artificial flavourings or colourings. Rooibosch tastes closest to 'ordinary' tea. Hot tomato juice makes a nice winter warmer. Roasted dandelion root 'coffee' (avoid added lactose) tastes good and is wonderful for detoxifying your liver.

☺ COLD DRINKS: filtered or bottled water, still or sparkling, with added ice and lemon not only looks good but is refreshing and delicious. (As an alternative to buying bottles of sparkling mineral water, use a filter jug and a soda siphon.) Chilled tomato juice (no citric acid or vinegar) is good as a 'starter', and iced fruit teas (no citric acid or malt!) make a tasty alternative to fruit juice in summer. Try whisking yoghurt with sparkling mineral water and adding mint or vanilla essence!

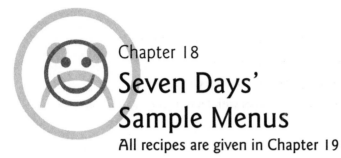

Chapter 18

Seven Days'
Sample Menus
All recipes are given in Chapter 19

DAY 1

Breakfast Porridge.

Lunch Home-made baked beans with soda bread and salad.

Dinner Tomato and tuna topping with wholewheat spaghetti or instant wholewheat noodles. Sliced green beans, fresh or frozen.

Dessert Yoghurt surprise.

DAY 2

Breakfast Muesli base with soya milk or natural yoghurt.

Lunch Hummus with oatcakes and crudités.

Dinner Piperade with veggie pile and new potatoes.

Dessert Creamy carob.

DAY 3

Breakfast Fish cakes.

Lunch Pizza scones with salad.

Dinner Bean and vegetable stew with brown rice.

Dessert Lemon cheesecake.

DAY 4

Breakfast Scrambled egg with soda bread toast.

Lunch Falafel, corn bread and salad.

Dinner Chicken risotto with a green vegetable.

Dessert Avocado pancakes with lemon and coconut sauce.

DAY 5

Breakfast Canned salmon, tomato, cucumber and oatcakes.

Lunch Chicken and tarragon burgers with soda bread rolls.

Dinner Aubergine quiche and salad with yoghurt dressing.

Dessert Lemon and carrot crumble.

DAY 6

Breakfast Crunchy breakfast cereal.

Lunch Lentil wedges with crudités and cottage cheese.

Dinner Poisson del mar with potato and parsnip bake.

Dessert Steamed pudding with baked egg custard.

DAY 7

Breakfast Pease pudding and tomatoes.

Lunch Kedgeree.

Dinner Baked lemon chicken breasts with baked chips and side salad.

Dessert Lemon and carrot crumble.

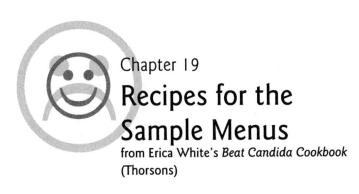

Chapter 19

Recipes for the Sample Menus

from Erica White's *Beat Candida Cookbook*
(Thorsons)

All the recipes are taken from the *Beat Candida Cookbook* and have a star rating to denote their simplicity or, put another way, the energy required to prepare them! For recipes requiring the least energy, the rating is one star (*). Basic baking and recipes using a moderate amount of energy have two stars (**). Meals in the *Cookbook* which could be served for dinner parties and take a fair amount of preparation have three stars (***), but none are included here because many of the * and ** recipes are quite delicious, and there is no point in expending unnecessary energy!

For people with specific food intolerances, e.g. wheat or even all the gluten grains, the *Cookbook* includes special sections giving advice and additional recipes, although many recipes throughout the book indicate that they are gluten-free.

BREAKFASTS

Oatmeal Porridge: Microwave Version *

Wheat-free, serves 2

My own favourite version of this is made with jumbo oats and soya milk, using level measures of each. This makes it really thick and creamy. Topped with a sprinkling of cinnamon, it's quite delicious!

1 cup porridge oats
2 cups water or soya milk (or half-and-half)
Optional: pinch of Lo-Salt

1 Cook, uncovered, on full power for 1½–2 minutes, stirring halfway through cooking time.
2 Serve with a little cold soya milk poured over, or with natural yoghurt stirred in.

Oatmeal Porridge: Saucepan Version *

It's almost as easy to make porridge in a saucepan, but you're left with a sticky pan to clean. Make sure you fill it with water as soon as you've poured the porridge!
Ingredients as for microwave version (above).

1 Heat in a saucepan, stirring all the time, and boil for one minute.

Muesli Base *

Muesli base is simply made up of your own mix of cereal flakes. Alternatively, you can buy it direct from a health-food store, but be careful to check it contains no dried fruits or nuts. Try the following mixture:

450g/1 lb/2 cups jumbo oats
350g/12oz/3 cups wheat flakes
350g/12oz/3 cups barley flakes
350g/12oz/3 cups rye flakes

Try throwing in a handful of any seeds you fancy – sunflower, sesame, pumpkin or linseeds. Keep it all in an airtight container.

Crunchy Breakfast Cereal **

You can also use muesli base to make a crunchy breakfast cereal.

350g/12oz/3 cups muesli base
50g/2oz/½ cup wheatgerm
50g/2oz/½ cup sunflower seeds
50g/2oz/½ cup sesame seeds
50g/2oz/½ cup desiccated coconut
4–5 tbsp extra virgin olive oil

1 Heat the oven to 350°F/180°C/Gas Mark 4. Mix together all the ingredients and spread on a large baking sheet. Bake for 45 minutes, stirring every 10–15 minutes.
2 Tip into another flat dish to cool before storing in an airtight container. Serve with natural yoghurt, or with hot or cold soya milk to provide protein.

Fish Cakes *

Gluten-free, serves 2

Fish cakes are good hot or cold for any meal, but you possibly hadn't considered them for breakfast. Using canned fish means they are particularly quick and easy to make. They may be frozen cooked or uncooked.

1 can pilchards or mackerel in brine
1 tbsp tomato purée (no citric acid)
1 small onion, finely chopped
½ mug soya flour
1 tsp dried mixed herbs

1 Drain and mash fish and combine well with all ingredients.
2 Make into burger shapes – 4 large or 6 medium. Grill for 5
   minutes each side, or fry in a little olive oil, turning after a few
   minutes, or bake in preheated oven at 400°F/200°C/Gas Mark
   6 for 30 minutes.

Scrambled Eggs: Microwave Version *

Gluten-free, serves 1 or 2

2 free-range eggs
2 tbsp soya milk
Freshly ground black pepper

1 Beat ingredients in a jug or bowl, and cook uncovered for
   about 2–2½ minutes, stirring every half-minute.

Scrambled Eggs: Saucepan Version *

Ingredients as for Microwave Version except that you need to
add a knob of unsalted butter.

1 Melt the butter in a saucepan and let it coat the bottom and
   sides before you add the mixture.
2 Beat eggs, soya milk and seasoning in a bowl and pour into
   the coated saucepan.
3 Cook over a low heat, stirring all the time, until set and creamy.
4 Serve on toasted soda bread or eat with rice cakes and
   unhydrogenated margarine.

Pease Pudding Slices with Tomato *

Grain-free, gluten-free, serves 2

1 can pease pudding
1–2 tomatoes, sliced
Freshly ground black pepper

1 Open both ends of the can and push pease pudding through.
   Cut into six thick slices.
2 Grill both sides then top with sliced tomatoes and continue
   to grill until tomatoes soften.
3 Serve sprinkled with pepper.

Alternatively, place sliced pease pudding and tomatoes on a
covered plate in the microwave. Don't heat too long unless you
like your tomatoes mushy!

Oatcakes **

Wheat-free

225g/8oz/2½ cups oats
50g/2oz/½ cup soya flour
2 tbsp sesame seeds
3 tbsp extra virgin olive oil
Boiling filtered water to mix

1 Preheat oven to 400°F/200°C/Gas Mark 6.
2 Combine oats, soya flour and sesame seeds. Rub in the oil.
3 Pour boiling water a little at a time, mixing to obtain a firm
   dough. Leave for a few moments to cool slightly.
4 Roll out and cut into shapes. Place on a non-stick tray and
   bake until golden.

LUNCHES

Quick Home-made Baked Beans *

Gluten-free

2 onions
1 tbsp extra virgin olive oil
400g/14oz can tomatoes (no citric acid)
2 tbsp tomato purée (no citric acid)
1 tsp mixed herbs and 1 tsp paprika
Freshly-ground black pepper
1 medium can haricot beans in salt water (sugar-free)

1 Finely chop onions and soften in oil over gentle heat. Add tomatoes, tomato purée, herbs, paprika and pepper. Stir well, mashing tomatoes, and simmer for a few minutes to obtain a fairly thick sauce. If you want it to be smooth, put it through a blender.
2 Drain and rinse the beans and add to the sauce.
3 Heat through, and serve in a baked potato or on toasted gluten-free soda bread. Can also be eaten cold with salad.

Yoghurt Soda Bread **

This basic bread recipe is a firm favourite, and many of my clients have produced variations on the theme. This will make two small loaves or one large one. If you want to make a batch for the freezer, a 1.5kg/3½lb bag of flour and a 1 litre/1¾ pint tub of yoghurt (with 6 tsp bicarbonate and ½ litre/¾ pint warm water) makes six small loaves.

450g/1 lb/3¼ cups wholewheat plain flour
2 tsp potassium (or sodium) bicarbonate
300ml/½pt/1½ cups natural yoghurt
150ml/¼ pint/⅔ cup warm water

1 Preheat the oven to 400°F/200°C/Gas Mark 6.
2 Sift the flour and mix in the raising agent, then stir in the
   yoghurt and warm water. Mix together well then coat the
   mixture with more flour and liberally flour your working
   surface. No kneading is necessary.
3 If making small loaves, divide mixture into two and make
   into fairly flat, oval shapes. Cut a cross on the top. Place on
   a floured tray and bake for 30 minutes, then turn oven down
   to 350°F/180°C/Gas Mark 4 for another 20 minutes.
4 To test if it's ready, tap the bottom of the loaf and it should
   sound hollow. Leave to cool on a wire rack. Six loaves in the
   oven might require a little more baking time.

Soda Bread Rolls **

Use the bread mixture to make small rolls. Cook for 20 minutes
at 400°F/200°C/Gas Mark 4. These are lovely eaten warm with
soup if your digestion is up to it!

Hummus *

Gluten-free

1 can sugar-free chickpeas (garbanzos), rinsed to remove salt
½–1 tsp garlic granules, according to preference
150ml/¼ pt/⅔ cup natural low-fat yoghurt
½ lemon, squeezed

1 Mix all ingredients in processor or blender; leave slightly
   lumpy. Keep refrigerated.

Crudités *

Many raw vegetables are suitable, e.g. carrots, celery, cucumber, cauliflower, peppers, radishes, swedes, mooli (long white radishes). You can cut some into matchsticks, some into rings or slices, and cauliflower of course makes pretty florets. Choose three or four with contrasting colours and use a variety of shapes.

Pizza Scones **

225g/8oz/1½ cups plain wholemeal flour
2 tsp potassium (or sodium) bicarbonate
50g/2oz/¼ cup unsalted butter
125ml/4 fl oz/½ cup soya milk
4 tsp fresh lemon juice

Topping:
1 tbsp extra virgin olive oil
1 medium onion, chopped
400g/4oz/2 cups canned tomatoes (no citric acid)
½ tsp mixed dried herbs

Extra topping ideas: prawns, tuna, cottage cheese, sweetcorn, green pepper, cooked chicken.

1 Preheat oven to 425°F/220°C/Gas Mark 7.
2 Sift dry ingredients and rub in butter. Add soya milk and lemon juice and mix to a soft dough.
3 Knead lightly on floured surface. Roll out to 12mm/½-inch thickness. Cut out 5cm/2½-inch rounds and place on floured baking sheet. Bake for 10–12 minutes.
4 While scones are baking, heat the oil in a pan, add the onion and cook gently until soft. Chop the tomatoes and add to pan together with herbs, and cook till sauce is reduced to jam-like consistency.

5 Remove scones from oven, cut in halves and put them back on the baking sheet, cut side up. Put a spoonful of mixture on each and spread it to the edges. Put on any extra toppings, then bake for a further 10-12 minutes.

Falafel *

Gluten-free

225g/8oz/1 cup chickpeas (garbanzos), soaked and cooked
    (or 1 medium can, sugar-free, rinsed)
1 free-range egg
1 onion, finely chopped
2 tbsp fresh parsley, chopped
1 clove garlic, crushed
1 tsp ground coriander
1 tsp ground cumin
Freshly ground black pepper
Buckwheat flour for moulding
2 tbsp extra virgin olive oil

1 Put all ingredients except buckwheat flour and oil into food processor and blend until mostly smooth. Mix with buckwheat flour to a consistency that will shape into patties.
2 Shallow fry in the oil for 3 minutes on each side. Stand on kitchen paper on a plate in a low oven to keep warm.
3 Serve with brown rice and salad.

Lentil Wedges *

Gluten-free

225g/8 oz/1 cup red lentils
450ml/¾ pint/2 cups water
1 large onion, diced
1 tbsp extra virgin olive oil
1 tsp dried mixed herbs
1 free range egg
Freshly ground black pepper

1 Preheat oven to 375°F/190°C/Gas Mark 5.
2 Cook the lentils in the water until soft and no liquid is left.
3 Sauté onion in oil until soft.
4 Combine all ingredients and press into a 22cm/9-inch sandwich tin lined with greaseproof paper. Bake for 30 minutes. Serve hot or cold.

Chicken and Tarragon Burgers *

May be wheat-free, makes 6

450g/1 lb/2 cups minced raw chicken
1 onion
Fresh tarragon, roughly chopped – as much as liked
85g/3oz/1 cup rolled oats
Flour for dusting – any type – wheat, rye, potato, gram or rice.

1 Mix the chicken, onion, tarragon and oats together until mixture does not cling to sides of the bowl. The mixture is moist so nothing should be needed to bind it.
2 Dust surface with flour and shape tablespoonsful of mixture into small round cakes about 8 cm/3 inches in diameter and 2-cm/¾-inch thick. Place on a greased baking tray and cook at

375°F/190°C/Gas Mark 5, turning regularly, for about 45
minutes or until insides look cooked.

3 Can be served with jacket potatoes and stir-fried vegetables,
or cold with a salad, or in a soda bread roll with home-made
tomato sauce if you are pining for a burger!

Kedgeree *

Gluten-free

Kedgeree has been one of my husband's favourite meals for
many years! Our offspring can remember having it as children in
seaside holiday cottages whenever it was Daddy's turn to cook!
It has the advantage of being able to use absolutely any type of
fish at all – baked white fish or a can of salmon or tuna or even
frozen prawns. My own preference is for freshly cooked white
fish, preferably haddock. You will soon find your own favourite,
and it is so easy to make.

450g/1 lb baked white fish (or can of tuna or salmon in brine
    or 225g/8oz/2 cups prawns)
Optional: 125g/4 oz/1 scant cup frozen green peas
125g/4 oz/⅔ cup brown rice
2 hard-boiled free-range eggs
2 tbsp fresh parsley or chives
Optional: ½ large can sweetcorn (sugar-free)
Segments of organic lemon

1 Cook the white fish or open and thoroughly drain the can of
tuna or salmon or defrost the prawns, if frozen.
2 Cook the green peas, if using.
3 Roughly flake the fish into fairly large pieces. Cook the brown
rice and when all the water has been taken up, mix in all the
other ingredients.
4 Serve with segments of lemon to squeeze over the top – and
enjoy it!

DINNERS

Tomato and Tuna Topping *

Gluten-free

This is quick and useful for serving on a baked potato or some wholemeal pasta – or on toasted wholemeal soda bread.

2 tsp tomato purée (no citric acid)
150ml/¼ pt/⅔ cup filtered water
1 small onion, chopped
200g/7oz can tuna in brine, drained
Pinch of dried oregano

1 Mix the tomato purée with the water in a saucepan. Add the onion and cook gently for a few minutes until soft.
2 Flake the tuna and add it to the mixture. Stir, add oregano, and continue cooking till thoroughly heated and the liquid has reduced a little.

Piperade *

Gluten-free, serves 2–4

The following recipe is rather like a Spanish omelette, but uses tomatoes rather than potatoes.

1 medium onion, finely chopped
2 cloves garlic, crushed (or 1 tsp garlic granules)
2 tbsp extra virgin olive oil
2 green or red peppers or mixed, deseeded and chopped
4 tomatoes, roughly chopped
6 free-range eggs
Fresh parsley, finely chopped

1 Soften the onion and garlic in the oil over a gentle heat for 5 minutes, then add the peppers and tomatoes for a further 5 minutes.
2 Beat the eggs in a separate bowl, then pour over the cooked vegetables and mix them in until lightly scrambled.
3 Garnish with parsley. Cut into required number of servings.

Veggie Pile *

Gluten-free

If you need a nutritious fill-up just for yourself, divide the quantities by four and use a small saucepan.

8 sticks celery, chopped
1 large green pepper, deseeded and cut into long slices
1 large red or yellow pepper, deseeded and cut into long slices
2 large courgettes (zucchini), sliced into rounds
Alternatives: sliced white cabbage is good

1 Put all the vegetables into a large saucepan or wok with a lid, with just a puddle of boiling water in the bottom. Boil fast for no more than four minutes, but take off the lid and stir a few times during cooking.

Bean and Vegetable Stew *

2 medium onions, chopped
1 green pepper, deseeded and chopped
4 large cups of any other vegetables, chopped
Water to cover
2 tbsp fine oatmeal mixed with 8 tbsp cold water
4 tbsp tomato purée (no citric acid)
1 tsp dried mixed herbs

2 cans of kidney or haricot beans or chickpeas (garbanzos) (no sugar)

1 Lightly cook the vegetables in water which just covers them.
2 When tender, mix the oatmeal and water in a bowl, then add some of the hot vegetable juice to it, stirring carefully.
3 When the paste is smooth, add it to the hot water with the vegetables, stirring all the time. Cook for two minutes, till the gravy is thick, then stir in the tomato purée and herbs.
4 Drain and thoroughly rinse the beans, then tip them in with the vegetables and heat through gently, making sure that the gravy doesn't 'catch' on the bottom.

Chicken Risotto **

Gluten-free

2 tbsp extra virgin olive oil
225g/8oz/1 cup brown rice
450g/1lb/2 cups chicken breast, cubed
125g/4 oz/1 scant cup carrot, diced
1 large onion, finely chopped
1 tsp paprika
1 tbsp tomato purée (no citric acid)
2 beef tomatoes, skinned and chopped
125ml/4 fl oz/½ cup water

1 Heat the oil in a deep pan and add half the rice, cooking for 3 minutes on low heat. Add the carrot and onion and cook for 3 more minutes.
2 Add the chicken and cook for 3 more minutes, stirring. Add everything else and stir. Simmer for 45 minutes or until the rice is cooked and all the liquid is absorbed.
3 Cook the remaining rice separately to serve with the risotto and a green vegetable.

Aubergine (Eggplant) Quiche *

*Basic Shortcrust Pastry ** (*)*
3 heaped tbsp plain wholemeal flour
2 heaped tbsp fine or medium oatmeal
2 tbsp unrefined sunflower oil
Filtered water to mix

Optional (for a softer pastry):
1 tsp potassium (or sodium) bicarbonate
2 tsp fresh lemon juice

1   Mix together the dry ingredients, and mix in the oil (and
    lemon juice, if optional bicarbonate powder is being used).
    Add water till you have a very sticky dough which just holds
    together. (In a processor, it suddenly forms a ball.)
2   Coat with plenty of flour for handling, but the wetter the
    dough the better. Roll out on a floured surface (roll more
    thinly if using bicarbonate powder).

*Blind-baked Quiche or Flan Case ***
This is done incredibly quickly in a microwave.

1   Make one measure of the basic shortcrust pastry, and roll it
    out to fit a 25cm/10-inch china or glassware flan dish.
2   Prick the bottom all over with a fork, then cover the centre
    with two pieces of kitchen roll and cover the edges with
    narrow strips of tinfoil (yes, tinfoil!).
3   Microwave on High for 4 minutes, remove the paper and foil
    and microwave again for 2 minutes. When you have put in
    the filling, you can either microwave on high for 10 minutes,
    or bake in a preheated oven at 350°F/180°C/Gas Mark 4 for
    30-40 minutes. Alternatively, you can blind-bake the case in
    the oven at the same temperature for 20 minutes before
    adding the filling and completing as before.

Gluten-free filling *
½ an aubergine (eggplant), diced
1 medium onion, chopped
2 tsp extra virgin olive oil
3 free-range eggs, beaten
300ml/½pt/1⅓ cups soya milk (or rice milk)

1 Preheat oven to 400°F/200°C/Gas Mark 6.
2 Lightly fry the aubergine (eggplant) and onion in the oil and
   put into pastry case.
3 Mix the eggs with the soya milk and pour on to vegetables.
4 Bake for 45 minutes, reducing heat to 300°F/150°C/Gas Mark
   2 for the last 30 minutes.

Poisson del Mar *

Gluten-free

This recipe has a definite continental flavour and is adapted from
the cookbook of a Bible College in France, where a client of mine
is based as a missionary. Although high in fat, its 'richness' is
counteracted by the large amount of lemon juice.

150g/5oz/⅔ cup unsalted butter (or 5 tbsp extra virgin olive oil)
2 large lemons, squeezed
1 large onion, diced
1 tsp fresh parsley, chopped
Freshly ground black pepper
Cod, haddock or halibut steaks, etc.

1 Preheat oven to 350°F/180°C/Gas Mark 4.
2 Melt the butter (or warm the oil) and mix with lemon juice
   and diced onion. Add chopped parsley and a shake of pepper.
3 Pour sauce over fish in an oiled or buttered dish. Bake for
   25–30 minutes.
4 Serve with brown rice.

Potato and Parsnip Bake *

450g/1 lb/3 cups potatoes, scrubbed
450g/1 lb/3 cups parsnips, scrubbed
4 tbsp fresh parsley, chopped
4 tbsp soda breadcrumbs

1 Preheat oven to 400°F/200°/Gas Mark 6.
2 Cook the potatoes and parsnips in a little filtered water till just done, then mash with a little of the cooking water, adding the parsley.
3 Lightly grease a baking tin (with butter or extra virgin olive oil), put the vegetables in and bake till crispy (30–40 minutes).
4 Remove from oven, top with breadcrumbs and return to oven to brown.

Baked Chips *

Gluten-free

This is an excellent way of making chips without fat, and there couldn't be an easier way of cooking potatoes – except perhaps baking them whole in their jackets.

1 Preheat oven to 375°F/190°C/Gas Mark 5.
2 Scrub two potatoes (peel or leave in skins), cut into 12mm/½-inch slices then cut through again to make chips. Arrange in a layer on an oiled or non-stick baking sheet and bake for 40–45 minutes.

Baked Lemon Chicken Breasts *

Gluten-free

You could bake jacket potatoes at the same time and serve them with cottage cheese and have a crisp green salad as a side dish.

2 organic lemons
4 chicken breasts, skinned

1 Scrub the lemons and grate the rinds, then squeeze out their juice.
2 Marinate the chicken breasts with the lemon juice and grated rind in a covered bowl overnight in the refrigerator.
3 Preheat oven to 375°F/190°C/Gas Mark 5.
4 Place chicken breasts on an oiled baking sheet and bake for ¾–1 hour, or until thoroughly cooked and golden.

DESSERTS

Yoghurt Surprise *

Serves 1 or 2

Small tub natural yoghurt
1 tbsp pumpkin seeds
1 tbsp sunflower seeds
1 tbsp linseeds
1 tbsp wheatgerm
Optional: 1 tbsp lecithin granules, 2 tbsp whole puffed rice

Mix together all the ingredients.

Creamy Carob Dessert **

Gluten-free

If this mixture is required as a filling, it can be blended in a liquidizer just before use to make it creamy rather than set.

3 × 42g/1½oz bars carob confection (dairy-free, sugar-free)
450ml/16 fl oz/ 2 cups soya milk (or rice milk)
½–1 tsp natural vanilla essence
1 tsp agar-agar
8 tbsp cold filtered water

1 Break up two carob bars into a basin and stand in a saucepan of hot water. Whilst melting, gently heat the soya milk then gradually pour onto the carob, stirring all the time. Add vanilla essence. When mixed together well, remove from heat.
2 Put agar-agar into the cold water in a saucepan and bring to the boil. When dissolved, allow to cool then stir into the carob mixture.
3 Pour through a sieve into a glass bowl or into individual glasses. Chill in refrigerator until set like blancmange then decorate top with grated carob from the other bar.

Lemon Cheesecake * & **

*Base ***
6 whole rye crispbreads
1 tbsp unsalted butter

1 Crush the crispbreads in a plastic bag, using a rolling pin.
2 Melt the butter in a saucepan and add the crumbs.
3 Press into the bottom of a buttered tin with a wooden spoon.

Lemon Cheesecake Topping **
450g/1 lb/2 cups cottage cheese
2 free-range eggs, separated
Juice of ½ lemon

1 Preheat oven to 350°F/180°C/Gas Mark 4.
2 Mix together the cheese, egg yolks and lemon juice.
3 Whisk the egg whites till stiff, fold into mixture with metal spoon.
4 Pour onto prepared base in tin, and bake for 40–45 minutes till slightly brown. Allow to cool. May be chilled in refrigerator or served at room temperature.

American Pancakes **

1 free-range egg
230ml/8 fl oz/1 cup natural yoghurt
1 tbsp fresh lemon juice
2 tbsp extra virgin olive oil
140g/5 oz/1 cup wholemeal flour
1 tsp potassium (or sodium) bicarbonate
Filtered water to mix

1 This mixture is very easily made by putting all ingredients together into a food processor. Otherwise, beat the egg, then add the yoghurt, lemon juice and olive oil, continuing to beat.
2 Sift the flour and bicarbonate powder and stir into the mixture, adding sufficient water to give a thick but liquid consistency.
3 Heat a griddle or a heavy-based frying pan, without oil. Drop spoonfuls of the mixture into the pan in smallish rounds, allowing room to spread. When the edges look done and bubbles pop up on the surface, they are ready to turn and cook for a further minute or two.

Lemon and Coconut Sauce *

Possibly the flavour we most associate with pancakes is lemon. In my family tradition, at least, lemon pancakes were always a tea-time treat on Shrove Tuesday. Here's a way of recapturing that particular memory.

3 lemons
3 tbsp desiccated coconut (or freshly-grated coconut)

1 Squeeze the lemons, put the juice in a blender with the coconut and liquidize. Otherwise, just stir well together.
2 Pour mixture onto each pancake, roll up and pour more over the top. Serve while the pancake is still hot.

Steamed Pudding **

Gluten-free, serves 1

Who says you can't have pudding at Christmas? This one is light and easy to digest, unlike the conventional Christmas pud.

60g/2½ oz/½ cup brown rice flour
40g/1½ oz/¼ cup maize meal
1 tsp carob powder
1 tsp potassium (or sodium) bicarbonate
1 small carrot, grated
2 tsp fresh lemon juice
30g/1½ oz/scant ¼ cup unhydrogenated margarine
4 tbsp soya milk (or rice milk)
Pinch each of ginger, nutmeg, cinnamon, mace

1 Mix all dry ingredients together in a bowl, stir in the grated carrot and add the lemon juice.

2 Gently melt the margarine with the milk and stir into the mixture in stages, stopping when the mixture is very soft but not runny.

3 Spoon into a greased pudding basin, cover with greaseproof paper and tie up with muslin. Place the basin in a saucepan with enough water to come two-thirds up the sides of the basin. Boil for 1 hour, topping up with boiling water as necessary, or cook in a steamer for the same time. A slow-cooker is an ideal way of cooking puddings because you can leave it all day or all night and forget about it.

Baked Egg Custard *

Gluten-free

3 free-range eggs, beaten
600ml/1 pint/2½ cups soya milk or rice milk
1–2 tsp natural vanilla essence, according to taste
Freshly grated nutmeg

1 Preheat oven to 325°F/170°C/Gas Mark 3.
2 Butter an oven-proof dish and put in the beaten eggs.
3 Warm the milk in a saucepan then pour it onto the eggs, stirring thoroughly. Add vanilla essence and sprinkle with nutmeg.
4 Put the dish into the oven, standing it on a baking tray which contains cold water. Bake for 40 minutes or until set.

Lemon and Carrot Crumble *

May be gluten-free

For many people, fruit crumble is a favourite pudding. This next good idea was sent in by Jonathan, who was obviously determined not to be deprived of something he likes so much!

1 organic lemon

125g/4 oz/1 scant cup wholewheat flour (or gluten-free flour,
  see below)

50g/2oz/¼ cup unsalted butter (or 4 tsp unrefined sunflower oil
  or extra virgin olive oil)

1 carrot

1 Preheat oven to 350°F/180°C/Gas Mark 4.
2 Scrub the lemon well, then grate the rind into a mixing bowl.
   Add the flour and butter or oil and rub together to form a
   crumble.
3 Take off the remaining lemon skin and cut the flesh into
   small pieces. Grate the carrot and place with the chopped
   lemon in an oven-proof dish with a small amount of water.
4 Place the crumble topping on top of the lemon and carrot
   and bake for 30 minutes.

Variations to filling: replace carrot with parsnip, sweet potato or
turnip; add desiccated coconut or a little cinnamon or nutmeg.

Variations to topping: add sesame seeds, coarse oatmeal or
oatflakes, rice flakes, millet flakes, etc. For a gluten-free version,
replace wheatflour with brown rice, buckwheat or maize flours.

Avocado Dessert *

Gluten-free, dairy-free

3 large carrots
3 large, ripe avocados
1 organic lemon
1 tsp ground cinnamon
Optional: 3 tbsp desiccated coconut
Few tbsp filtered water (or organic carrot juice, no citric acid)
Sesame seeds (optional)

1 Peel carrots, chop or grate and put in food processor. Add flesh of avocados, zest and juice of lemon, cinnamon (and coconut if desired) and water and blend until a thick 'fool' consistency is achieved, adding more water if necessary. Carrot juice instead of water gives an interesting variation in flavour.
2 Pour into container with lid and refrigerate. Keeps up to 3 days. May be sprinkled with sesame seeds for variety.

And for good measure, here are some cakes to help fill you up!

If you have a food processor, any of the following recipes would obviously be easier to make and could even be given a * rating.

Basic Carrot Cake ** (*)

1 free-range egg
4 tbsp unsalted butter
2 cups grated carrot
250g/8oz/1½ cups plain wholemeal flour
1 tsp potassium (or sodium) bicarbonate
½ tsp ground cinnamon
2 tsp fresh lemon juice
Soya milk (or rice milk) to mix

1 Preheat oven to 325°F/160°C/Gas Mark 3.
2 Beat together the egg and butter then fold in the grated carrot.
3 Sift together the dry ingredients and mix in well.
4 Add lemon juice and soya or rice milk till mixture just drops off the spoon. Pour into loaf tin which has been brushed with olive oil or melted butter and bake for 1 hour.
5 Allow to stand a little, then turn out carefully onto a wire rack to cool.

Ginger Cake (or Ginger and Walnut) ** (*)

125g/4 oz/½ cup unsalted butter
2 free-range eggs
2½ tsp ground ginger
150g/5oz/1 cup plain wholemeal flour
1 tsp potassium (or sodium) bicarbonate
2 tsp fresh lemon juice
Optional: 50g/2 oz freshly cracked chopped walnuts

1 Preheat oven to 400°F/200°C/Gas Mark 6.
2 Cream the butter and eggs then sift the ginger with the flour
   and bicarbonate powder and add to mixture in the bowl.
3 Add lemon juice, then the chopped walnuts if using, saving
   some pieces for the top.
4 Bake in a lined sandwich tin for 20 minutes.

Carob Crunchies *

May be gluten-free

50g/2oz/⅓ cup carob confection bar (dairy-free, sugar-free),
   broken in squares
2 cups whole-grain puffed rice (or whole-grain wheatflakes
   or puffed wheat)
Optional: 2 tbsp desiccated coconut
Fairy cake cases

1 Melt carob bar in a bowl over a saucepan of boiling water.
2 Tip in the other ingredients and mix thoroughly till cereals
   are covered.
3 Put into fairy cake cases, and set in refrigerator.

The following two recipes are enjoyable with a scraping of unsalted
butter or unhydrogenated margarine.

Rye Slice *

75g/3oz/½ cup wholewheat flour
75g/3oz/½ cup rye flour
75g/3oz/½ cup barley flour
75g/3oz/½ cup soya flour
115g/4oz/1 cup rye flakes
3 tsp mixed spice
3 tbsp extra virgin olive oil
Boiling filtered water to mix

1 Preheat oven to 375°F/190°C/Gas Mark 5.
2 Combine flours, flakes and spice and rub or stir in the oil.
   Pour on boiling water slowly, mixing to form a dough.
3 Place into an oiled loaf tin and bake for 30–40 minutes.
   Alternatively, put into a suitable container and cook in the
   microwave on High for 6 minutes (600W). Cool on a rack.
   Serve sliced.

Blackcurrant Tea Loaf **

550g/1¼ lb/4 cups plain wholewheat flour
225g/8 oz/1½ cups brown rice flour
2 tsp potassium (or sodium) bicarbonate
2 large carrots, grated
350ml/12 fl oz/1½ cups blackcurrant herb tea (use 3 teabags), warm
3 tsp natural vanilla essence
4 tsp fresh lemon juice
1 large tub natural yoghurt

1 Preheat oven to 400°F/200°C/Gas Mark 6.
2 Mix dry ingredients, then stir in grated carrot.
3 Mix in blackcurrant tea, vanilla essence and lemon juice.
   Stir in yoghurt – the mixture should be quite moist.

4 Pour into lined tins and bake for 20 minutes at high
   temperature, then turn tins and bake for a further 20 minutes
   at reduced temperature (350°F/180°C/Gas Mark 4).

Corn Cakes **

Gluten-free

125g/4 oz/1 scant cup brown rice flour
165g/5½ oz/1 cup fine maize meal
2 tsp potassium (or sodium) bicarbonate
65g/2½ oz/⅓ cup unsalted butter (or 2½ tbsp unrefined sunflower oil)
240ml/8 fl oz/1 cup soya milk (or rice milk)
1 free-range egg
4 tsp fresh lemon juice

1 Preheat oven to 400°F/200°C/Gas Mark 6.
2 Sift together dry ingredients and rub in butter or oil.
3 Beat together soya milk, egg and lemon juice and stir into
   flour mixture.
4 Turn into a slightly greased 20cm/8-inch square baking tin
   and bake for 25 minutes. Test with a knife in the centre.
5 Cut into 5cm/2-inch squares and serve warm with a spread.

Carob Cake ** (*)

225g/8 oz/1½ cups plain wholemeal flour
1½ tsp potassium (or sodium) bicarbonate
3 tbsp carob powder
125g/4 oz/1½ cups oats
225g/8 oz/1 cup unsalted butter
150ml/¼ pt/⅔ cup soya milk (or rice milk)
3 tsp fresh lemon juice
1–2 tsp natural vanilla essence

1 Preheat oven to 375°F/190°C/Gas Mark 5.
2 Sift flour with bicarbonate and carob powder and add the
   oats.
3 Melt butter and mix with soya milk, lemon juice and vanilla
   essence, then add to flour mixture, stirring.
4 Bake in a lined tin for 45 minutes and leave in tin till quite
   cool.

Now it only remains for me to wish you well as you start to eat
your way to health. I hope you enjoy the recipes!

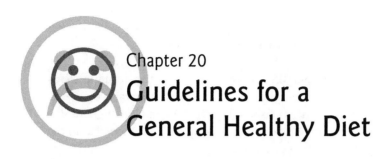

Chapter 20

Guidelines for a General Healthy Diet

The following eating plan is to show you what to aim for in a general, healthy diet. It will almost certainly not be specific enough to help you overcome major health problems such as arthritis or candidiasis but, once you are well, by following these guidelines your body will continue to function efficiently and so keep you in the best possible health.

So, if you are about to launch into a nutritional programme to help you overthrow a fatigue syndrome and if, as part of that plan, you will be following the anti-candida diet as described in Chapter 17 (as almost certainly you will need to), reading through the following guidelines will show you ways in which you will be able to relax that diet in due course, once you are well and have established a new healthy balance of microbes in your intestines.

Meanwhile, why not try to steer your family and friends towards the following healthy eating habits so that, if they are fortunate enough to be in good health, they may stay that way, or if they need help with improving energy and immunity, for instance, that they will find it by making some really quite simple changes to their eating habits.

1 At least half of your diet should consist of alkaline-forming foods, i.e., all vegetables, sprouted seeds, yoghurt (natural unsweetened), buckwheat, and freshly-cracked almonds.

2 The rest of your diet should consist of acid-forming foods such as whole grains, pulses, nuts (freshly cracked), seeds, eggs, cottage cheese, fish and poultry. Avoid refined grains like white flour and white rice as these quickly turn to sugar in the blood and have been depleted of many beneficial nutrients and fibre, causing an imbalance of vitamins and minerals and encouraging constipation.

3 Eat as much raw food as possible. Cooking destroys vitamins and breaks down the fibre in food. Have a large plate of salad at least once a day.

4 The best proportion of food at *every* meal and *every* snack is **one-third** good quality protein (fish, chicken, yoghurt, cottage cheese, beans, pulses, tofu) to **two-thirds** complex carbohydrates (all vegetables, fruits and whole grains). This gives you the best energy and the most efficient metabolism by helping to regulate blood sugar, support your adrenals and strengthen immunity.

5 Avoid sugar and other foods with concentrated sweetness. Honey and maple syrup are marginally better, but too sweet for people with a candida problem or low blood sugar! Dilute fruit juice 50/50 and soak dried fruit overnight. Many recipes using dried fruit, such as fruit cakes and Christmas puddings, you will find are sweet enough without adding sugar. Read labels and avoid products with unnecessarily-added sugar like tinned beans, tinned sweetcorn, frozen peas, tomato ketchup, etc., and be aware of all the words which simply indicate a form of sugar! These include sucrose, maltose, fructose, dextrose, lactose, glucose and syrup.

6 When using oils other than for cooking (i.e. for salad dressings, spreads, mayonnaise), use cold-pressed (or unrefined) sunflower, sesame, safflower or flax (linseed) oils. Do **not** use margarine which states 'Hydrogenated', even if it also claims to be high in polyunsaturates! The process of hydrogenation makes the oils more harmful to the body than saturated animal fats, so look for the word 'Unhydrogenated' on the tub before you buy it. The best oils produce prostaglandins which are needed for healthy hormonal function and skin health. They also reduce inflammation.

7 Avoid frying; grill or bake instead. If you do fry, use cold-pressed (unrefined or 'virgin') olive oil or a small amount of butter (which is actually safer at very high temperatures than sunflower oil!) and cook for as short a time as possible. Cold-pressed sunflower oil may be used at baking temperatures (it makes excellent pastry!) but it is damaging if used at higher temperatures.

8 Increase fish and poultry (free-range, to avoid antibiotics and hormones). Reduce red meats like beef, pork, lamb, ham and other high-fat foods. Even lean meat is 75 per cent fat. Among other things, they cause inflammation and so encourage aches and pains.

9 Increase vegetarian sources of protein. A complete protein is made by having a meal which combines *a grain* with *a pulse,* like spaghetti bolognese made with brown lentils in an onion and tomato sauce flavoured with herbs and eaten with wholewheat pasta (or corn pasta or rice pasta). Another idea is bean and vegetable pie, made with beans or chickpeas mixed with any type of vegetables and covered with a crumble topping or wholemeal pastry. (A good pastry mix is made with wholewheat flour, fine oatmeal and unrefined sunflower oil in

proportions of 3:2:2, with plenty of water and then dusted with plenty of flour). Both examples provide a meal which combines a grain with a pulse, the best possible food combination for protein value.

10 The essential fatty acid from oily fish is good for you, producing prostaglandins (hormone-like substances) which are beneficial for the health of your heart and arteries and so can help to reduce high blood pressure. They also reduce inflammation in the body. You get the same benefits from linseed (flax seeds). Another type of essential fatty acid is found in evening primrose oil and borage and also in various seeds – pumpkin, sunflower and sesame. It helps to correct hormonal imbalances, does marvels for your skin and is also anti-inflammatory.

11 The ideal intake of water is about 2 litres daily. However, a diet which has plenty of fruit and vegetables can supply almost half of this, since these foods are 90 per cent water. We should therefore aim at drinking 1 litre of water a day, taken as filtered or mineral water or in diluted fruit juice or herb or fruit teas.

12 Avoid foods with added salt. Don't add salt to your cooking and, if you must add something at the table, use Lo-Salt, which has more potassium than sodium. If you think your food lacks flavour without salt, this probably means that your body is zinc-deficient.

13 Avoid artificial additives and preservatives, which means avoiding most processed or 'fast' foods. Also avoid artificial sweeteners; they upset the chemical balance of the body and can even cause depression. In any case, they keep your sweet tooth alive, and that is something you are better without!

14 Avoid regular consumption of tea or coffee, preferably give them up completely! Caffeine is an addictive stimulant which plays havoc with your blood sugar levels and can cause emotional problems like depression and anxiety as well as physical problems like palpitations, migraine, insomnia, irritable bowel and cystitis. It also depletes the body of important minerals. Even decaffeinated products still contain other stimulants. Barleycup is a good alternative to coffee and Rooibosch is very like ordinary tea but without the harmful stimulants. There are many herbal and fruit teas to try. Roasted dandelion root makes a very pleasant alternative to coffee and is excellent at helping to detoxify the liver. You should also avoid cola drinks and Lucozade because they contain caffeine, as do some painkillers like Anadin. Chocolate contains some of the same stimulant drugs as tea and coffee, which is why it can be so addictive!

15 On average, if you want to drink some alcohol, don't drink more than one glass of wine, spirits or beer a day – and none at all if you have candida or low blood sugar or an intolerance to alcohol. Sparkling mineral water with ice and a slice of lemon is delicious and refreshing. Make some strong fruit tea using two teabags at a time and then chill and serve with ice to make a variety of different flavoured drinks.

16 And remember – smoking not only causes damage to your lungs and arteries but directly interferes with the absorption of many nutrients, causing nutritional deficiencies and imbalances which give rise to other health problems.

223

Part (5)

Choose Life!

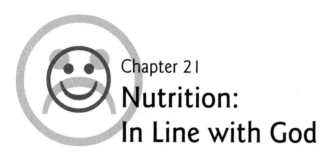

Chapter 21
Nutrition:
In Line with God

Life in a Fallen World

None of the problems associated with pollution, pesticides and depleted and adulterated foods existed when God first created man and put him on planet Earth, neither did they exist when Jesus lived in Galilee. Most of them didn't exist even as recently as the first half of the 20th century!

With increasing scientific knowledge and skill, mankind has managed to mess up his environment and his food. As a result, malnutrition is not confined to the Third World countries, as we tend to suppose, and the health of the Western world is spiralling downwards. A great many health problems are now accepted as being a normal part of life – yet simply do not occur when the body is optimally nourished.

For example, I have found that the majority of women expect to suffer monthly premenstrual miseries, yet I have also found over and over again that when diets are improved and nutritional deficiencies and imbalances have been corrected, the same women who regularly dissolved into tears or screamed at their husbands and children for a part of every month (and felt guilty the rest of the time!) now do not even notice their period starting and are able to remain the affectionate wives and mothers they really are. The accepted monthly trauma does not *need* to happen, and *will* not happen if women will only learn to take care of their hormones by returning as closely as possible to the original eating plan that was designed in order to put good fuel into our bodies' machinery, and by doing everything they possibly can to offset the damaging effects of environmental pollution.

They need to realize that it's the coffee they drink to keep them going (or the chocolate bars grabbed between meals, or the left-over cake finished up as they clear the table), together with a general lack of good nutritious food, which is actually causing them to feel and behave the way they do.

Getting to Grips

We need to get to grips with the situation, and, as a Christian myself, I believe that Christians should take a lead in this! It has been quite clear in my own life that God wanted me to understand the importance of being a proper 'steward' of my body, learning to treat it with the respect it deserves. Whatever I might think of it when I look in the mirror, it is in fact a quite amazing piece of handiwork! According to the Bible, it is also a temple of the Holy Spirit (1 Corinthians 3:16).

My experience of sickness into health enabled my body, as well as my soul and my spirit, to come into line with the truth of God's word in the Bible when it says, *'Through his wounds you have been healed'* (1 Peter 2:24). God's healing is given by grace (in other words, he freely gives us what we don't deserve and haven't had to earn), but that does not excuse us from living a life of faith and obedience.

When I reflect on what has happened in my life and consider how many Christians are now being led to contact me for nutritional advice, I cannot help but see God's hand in it all. It is also no accident that you are reading this book – at least, if you believe that God guides our lives, as I do. So what do you think is the purpose behind it?

Perhaps God wants to help you take hold of healing for your-self – or for someone near to you – through a nutritional approach like the one outlined in earlier chapters. I firmly believe (and hope you do, too) that God can heal in an instant if he chooses, yet for some reason there are times when he apparently decides to heal us through encouraging us to change our diet and take some vitamins!

Why should this be? Is it because he knows we need more self-discipline? That was definitely a need in my own life, and keeping to a strict diet certainly increases self-control! What better motivation could you have for doing it than knowing that it will not only help you to become well but that it is providing you with a way of pleasing God?

Perhaps there is a challenge for you; do you really *want* to be well? This might seem a ridiculous question, but Jesus once asked it of a man who had been ill for 38 years, so he must have known that sometimes it needs to be asked (John 5:6). When Jesus heard the faith in his reply, that man was healed 'at once', the Bible says!

If Jesus asked you the same question, is it possible that you might reply, 'Lord, you *know* I want to be well, but I couldn't possibly give up eating bread, or drinking tea, or eating chocolate . . .' or whatever else it might take to restore you to health?

He asks again, '*Do you **want** to be well?*'

Perhaps he wants you to trust him more for your needs? Food supplements – and, I'm afraid, professional advice – cost money. If you believe that God is leading you to nutritional help for your healing, should you really be saying, 'Oh, but I couldn't afford it!'? I have seen many times how he undertakes the financial cost for someone who looks to him for provision, confirming in the process that this is the way he has chosen for their healing. (Here I will say that there was a time when everything I recommended in a supplement programme for a UK client could be obtained on a National Health Service prescription if their doctor was willing to co-operate, but Government cuts have led to very few items indeed now being prescribable in this way. Although this is tragic, God will have a way for you to afford all that he wants you to have. I say this because he never asks us to do something without also giving us the resources to do it!)

Possibly God simply wants you to learn about the importance of good nutrition, so that your future life can be lived in health and not in constant need of healing. Is he concerned that you should think more responsibly about the food you feed to your family, so that the breadwinner doesn't keel over with a sudden heart attack, a teenage daughter doesn't succumb to anorexia and an elderly mother fall prey to brittle bones or senile dementia? So much can be done nutritionally to avoid each of these tragic situations. And for women approaching menopause, do you really think God intended that this stage of life should need the help of some artificial hormones?

Can we, before God, put our heads in the sand and do nothing about improving our own health and that of our families, simply because we don't want to give up eating the foods we like or deprive our families of the things they have grown to enjoy?

Perhaps you have thought it makes no difference whether you eat brown bread or white. Possibly, even, you have laughed at those who will eat only brown! But wouldn't you really rather eat the sort of wholesome food that Jesus ate? There would have been no white bread in Galilee 2,000 years ago, but for us it has become a main ingredient of our diet – yet white bread is of no value to our bodies; in fact it is decidedly harmful! Food is meant to do us good, not fill us with rubbish and man-made chemicals and additives.

God said, '*See, I give you all the seed-bearing plants that are upon the whole earth, and all the trees with seed-bearing fruit; this shall be your food.*' (Genesis 1:29)

He also said, '*Every living and crawling thing shall provide food for you, no less than the foliage of plants.*' (Genesis 9:3)

He provided us with good things to eat, and nowhere did he say, 'Go and mix up some chemicals to add to it, and refine the flour to remove its goodness'!

In Line with God's Wishes

I believe that, as Christians, we need to realize how much we have abused our bodies so that we can ask forgiveness and then learn anew how to live in ways which are pleasing to God. We will then be co-operating with him for the physical part of that fullness of life which Jesus has promised us (John 10:10), and our bodies will be submitted to him in the same way as our spirits and our minds.

The apostle John, writing to his friend Gaius, said, *'Dear friend, I am praying that all is well with you and that your body is as healthy as I know your soul is'* (3 John 1:2, Living Bible). John would never have prayed for something that was not in line with God's wishes; our Father *wants* us to be healthy!

Love God; honour and obey him in every way you can. Love your neighbour; let him see you radiating joy and peace and well-being, physical and mental as well as spiritual, then tell him how he can be the same – at every level! Love yourself and your family; show it by changing your shopping habits, start to read labels, learn all you can about healthy food and re-think your lifestyle to include relaxation and exercise. Ask God to help you with these everyday decisions. Invite him into your radical re-think. I am certain he will show you what he wants you to do! And when he makes it clear, show him your love and gratitude by doing what he asks.

Read this promise and claim it for yourself, as I did:

The Lord will keep all sickness far from you; he will not afflict you with those evil plagues of Egypt which you have known. (Deuteronomy 7:15, Jerusalem Bible)

But there is a condition for this promise which, if you read the preceding verses, you will find is wrapped up in just one word: obedience.

People sometimes argue that we all have to die some time, so there seems little point in denying ourselves the foods we enjoy just in case they happen to make us ill. I hope you agree with me that this attitude is hardly worth the paper it is printed on! Of course we shall die; nothing is more certain! But death does not have to come through sickness and pain. It should happen simply because our Father has called us home. Many of us have known elderly relatives who have somehow recognized their time to go, peacefully accepted it, and then just fallen asleep – to wake in a better place! And that's how I believe it is meant to be.

Meanwhile, we are meant to live life in all its fullness!

Attitudes and Choices

I believe that God is challenging all Christians about their attitudes to food. At the very least, he is wanting to sharpen up our self-control. Without realizing it, we eat for our own pleasure, for self-gratification, even though we might have given every other area of our lives to God for *his* pleasure. Fasting is encouraged in the Bible, but exercising control over the amount and type of food we eat can actually be harder to do than a total fast!

In addition, I believe God wants us to use our renewed minds (Romans 12:2) to make proper choices so that our bodies also might be renewed. The trouble is that this generation, through increased advertising and packaging pressure from the food industry, has come to regard as 'normal' whichever foods have the longest shelf-life, the greatest visual appeal, or the most addictive contents. There is nothing normal about such foods, except in the sense that they are eaten by the greatest number of people for the greater part of the time!

So What *Should* We Eat?

You really don't need me to tell you that the foods which are best for you are those which are completely natural, as God intended – fresh fruit and vegetables, whole grains made into delicious bread and pastry, many kinds of beans and pulses, nuts and seeds, eggs, low-fat dairy produce – and, unless you are a vegetarian, organic lean meat (which has not been adulterated with hormones, antibiotics and colouring), free-range poultry and any type of fish.

Why should those who eat food out of packets and quench their thirst out of cans be scornful of those who choose to eat *proper* food, knowing that this is the fuel which was specially designed for our bodies? As television advertising makes an increasing impact, isn't it time that Christians took a stand and refused to have their thinking and their spending moulded by the world? Paul says. *'Let your behaviour change, modelled by your new mind. This is the only way to discover the will of God and know what is good, what it is that God wants, what is the perfect thing to do'.* (Romans 12:2, Jerusalem Bible)

Very often people say, 'I'm a great believer in having a little of what you fancy! I can't cope with the idea of watching what I eat. Anyway, I'm never ill, so why should I bother?'

They somehow manage to say it with a fair degree of pride, as though they themselves are responsible for this happy state of affairs! They should instead praise God that he is keeping them healthy and that, as yet, he has not asked them to exercise more self-discipline. In any case, the situation will probably not continue all their lives because, after all, machinery is machinery and will not run indefinitely on low-grade fuel. It will either slow down and need lots of servicing, or else it will come to a sudden grinding halt! Unexpected heart attacks or strokes can happen largely because the diet has been deficient in magnesium, which is needed to enable muscles to relax after contracting. If muscles around the heart or an artery go into spasm, and there is not enough magnesium available to relax them, the consequences will be dire.

Magnesium is found in most dark green leafy vegetables (not spinach), dried fruit, some fresh fruit, nuts, seeds, whole grains – in other words, many of the foods which go to make a healthy diet. However, if too much calcium is supplied (from many of the same sources but also from milk products), the balance is tipped and muscles will more easily contract than relax. Too much cheese and other milky products alongside too few green vegetables, nuts and seeds could well lead to a scenario of muscle spasm blocking oxygen supply to the heart or brain. Some diet-related diseases give gradual warnings; with others there is no second chance.

Healing or Health?

Another opinion frequently expressed is that God would prefer to heal through prayer than through alternative therapies. My view is that God is God and will no doubt heal as he chooses! In any case, good nutrition should not be regarded as an alternative therapy. We are not talking about medicine, either orthodox or alternative, although the biochemical understanding of nutrition is in line with 'straight' Western medicine. We are talking about *food*. God might ask us to fast occasionally, but most of the time he expects us to eat! So although I agree that he is more than willing to heal through prayer or Christian ministry, I also believe that he would rather we learned how to be healthy.

It was a wonderful idea on God's part to give us delicious food as fuel rather than a smelly substance like petrol! Vitamin and mineral supplements are just a way of taking food in concentrated form when our bodies need some extra help. It would be great if they were not necessary, but unfortunately in these days of heavy pollution (when even organically grown vegetables contain harmful chemicals from the soil, carried there by contaminated rain) and adulterated food, our bodies need every bit of help they can get to cope with the situation and stay strong.

In some ways it did more harm than good when scientists identified the specific vitamins and minerals present in food, because many people then thought (and still do!) that they could continue with their bad diet and make up for it by taking some vitamin pills. *Nothing* can make up for a poor diet if we want to keep or regain our health.

For more than 40 years I ate a diet high in sugar, fat, stimulants and refined grains, with devastating consequences. Within a comparatively short time of realizing what I had been doing to myself and radically rethinking my eating habits, I came into a life so 'abundant' that sometimes I say, 'Oh, Lord, does it have to be *this* full?' – but he knows I'm only joking! In truth, how can I help but rejoice in my new-found stamina, which has given me better health at 65 years old than I had at 25 – or even 5!

Jesus once healed a blind man who later said, when questioned, '*I only know that I was blind and now I can see*' (John 9:25). I can identify with that, both in terms of previously blinkered understanding and of blighted health. But now I can see!

When I discovered that I was suffering from yeast infection, I received the laying-on of hands several times from faith-filled Christians who prayed that I might be healed of this specific illness. Each time I received an assurance that the healing *would* come, but that it would be in God's good time and so till then I had to trust him. I firmly believe that he could have healed me on the spot on any of those occasions, but he chose to heal me through a longer process that involved teaching me the importance of good nutrition.

God is a God of love and mercy and he has supernatural ability to heal, but I believe that he also asks us to take responsibility for those areas of our lives which he has entrusted to us, which includes our physical bodies. For why should he heal a man of lung cancer who refuses to give up smoking? And why should he heal a woman of obesity and heart disease if her daily food consists of fish and chips, pizza and burgers, with ice-cream and doughnuts to follow, and coffee, tea or cola to wash it all down?!

Outsmarting the Enemy!

By hearing what God is saying in these days of increasing pollution and undermined bodily defences, we can give the enemy less opportunity to invade our bodies with sickness and disease. We know that he will do whatever he can to make us ineffective as Christian witnesses and, although peace and patience from God can often be seen in one who is suffering, the sickness itself does nothing at all for God's glory and honour.

When I realized that our enemy the devil wages warfare against us, I was glad to discover the armour which God provides for our protection (Ephesians 6:10–16). By beginning to co-operate with God in taking care of my body, I made a stand against the enemy's tactics in the physical realm. That second helping of pudding or 'just one more' chocolate biscuit are probably the most common temptations most of us ever have to withstand in our ordinary, everyday lives. It is no coincidence that man's very first sin was to eat a tempting piece of forbidden fruit! The pleasure we derive from food plays an enormous part in our lives, and the devil knows what he is doing. For one thing, he knows it is much harder for us to fight once he has already weakened our bodies, and it even becomes a battle to pray when we are in the grips of pain or sickness.

Let us determine to thwart the enemy's attempts to ruin our lives and make us ineffective as Christians. Illness is no witness to God's love and power. If that's all you get for being a

Christian, who wants to know?

But Jesus says, '*Do you want to be well?*'

Do You Want to be Well?

Do you?

If so, and you put your faith in Jesus and do whatever he asks you to do, then the Bible promises that he will heal you. Whether your healing comes quickly as a supernatural answer to prayer, or whether it comes slowly as you obey him and persevere, the outcome is equally sure and the glory will go to God!

I have no desire to build false hopes in you. *I* do not make these promises. They are spoken by Jesus Christ himself.

Whatever you ask in my name, believe that you have received it, and it will be yours. (Mark 11:24)

Why don't you try believing him?

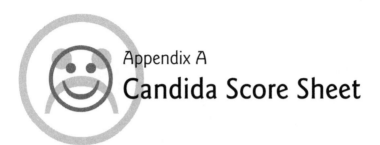

Appendix A
Candida Score Sheet

This Candida score will help you to assess the possibility or severity of yeast-related health problems

Risk factors:

1 Have you ever taken antibiotics for longer than a month or more than once in a year? .... If so, score 5 ......

2 Have you had a high-sugar diet, now or in the past – even as a child? Or have you ever lived through a high level of stress? .... If so, score 5 ......

3 Have you ever had a high alcohol intake, or taken drugs? .... If so, score 5 ......

4 Have you ever had any steroid treatments – pills, injections, creams, inhalers? (For women, this includes the contraceptive pill or hormone therapy) .... If so, score 10 ......

Present symptoms:

Score 1 point per line if any or all of the symptoms are occasional or mild.

Score 2 points per line if any or all of the symptoms are frequent or moderately severe.

Score 3 points per line if any or all of the symptoms are really severe or disabling.

(Score 1–3)

5 Depression, anxiety, irritability, mood swings ....

6 Poor memory, lack of concentration, feeling spacey or unreal.. ....

7 Fatigue, lethargy, feeling drained ....

8 Indigestion, heartburn, food intolerance, bloating, intestinal gas ....

9 Constipation, diarrhoea, irritable bowel syndrome, stomach ache, mucus in stools ....

10 *In women*: Premenstrual syndrome, period pain or irregularities, infertility, endometriosis, loss of sex drive ....

In men: Prostate problems, infertility, impotence, loss of sex drive ....

11 *In women*: Vaginal burning, itching, discharge ....

In men: Irritation of groin or genitals ....

12 Muscle aches or weakness, joint pain or stiffness... ....

13 Eczema, psoriasis, rashes, itching ....

14 Athlete's foot, ringworm, fungal toenails.............. ....

15 Cravings for sweet foods, chocolate, alcohol, bread ....

16 Sensitivity to perfume, chemical smells, petrol fumes, tobacco smoke ....

17 Any symptoms made worse on damp days
   or in mouldy places ....

18 Dizziness, loss of balance, recurrent ear
   infections, deafness ....

19 Insomnia, waking unrefreshed, drowsy
   during the day, need for excessive sleep ....

20 Body odour, bad breath ....

21 Sores in mouth, sore throat............................ ....

22 Nasal congestion, catarrh, sinusitis ....

23 Pain or tightness in chest, wheezing or
   shortness of breath ....

24 Urinary frequency, urgency, burning.................... ....

25 Spots in front of eyes, burning or watery eyes ....

26 Easy bruising, chilliness, cold hands and feet....... ....

27 Headache, migraine ....

28 Numbness, burning, tingling, incoordination ....

29 Irritation around anus ....

Total score   ....

Total score 75–100 – There is very little doubt that you have
yeast infection.
Total score 50–75 – You very probably have yeast infection.
Total score 25–50 – You quite possibly have yeast infection.
Total score 0–25 – Count yourself blessed – but watch your step!

Please note that this questionnaire is not as detailed as one
which might be used by a nutritional therapist, and which
therefore might give you a higher score. It is simply intended as
a guideline.

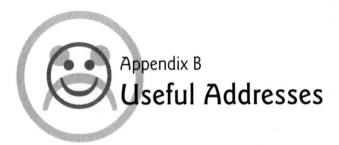

Appendix B
Useful Addresses

Diagnostic laboratories referred to in the text

Great Smokies Diagnostic Laboratory
63 Zillicoa Street
Asheville NC 28801–1074
USA
Telephone: 800-522-4762
e-mail: cs@gsdl.com
www.greatsmokies-lab.com

UK contact:
Health Interlink Ltd
Interlink House
1A Crown Street
Redbourn
Herts AL3 7JX
Telephone: 01582 794094
Fax: 01582 794909

The Great Plains Laboratory
9335 W. 75th Street
Overland Park
KS 66204
USA
Telephone: 913 341 8949
Fax: 913 341 6207
e-mail: williamsha@aol.com
www.autism.com/shaw-yeast

UK contact:
Health Interlink Ltd.
(details on previous page)

Diagnos-Techs, Inc
Clinical & Research Laboratory
PO Box 58948
Seattle
WA 98138-1948
Telephone: 425 251 0596

UK contact:
Diagnostech Ltd
Telephone: 0179 246 5492

BioMed International
55 Queens Road
East Grinstead
Sussex RH19 1BG
UK
Telephone: 01342 322854

Some Reputable Supplement Suppliers

UK

BioCare Ltd
Lakeside
180 Lifford Lane
Kings Norton
Birmingham
B30 3NU
Telephone: 44 (0) 121 433 3727 (Sales & General Enquiries)
Fax: 44 (0) 121 433 3879 (General Enquiries)
e-mail: biocare@biocare.co.uk

Nature's Best
1 Lamberts Road
Tunbridge Wells
TN2 3BE
Telephone: 44 (0) 1892 552117
Fax: 44 (0) 1892 515863

USA

Solgar Vitamin and Herb Company
500 Willow Tree Road
Leonia
New Jersey 07605
USA
www.solgar.com

Vital Life
Klaire Laboratories
1573 West Seminole
San Marcos
California 92069
USA
Telephone: (760) 744 9680

Thorne Research
25820 Highway 2 West
P.O. Box 25
Dover
Idaho 83825
USA
Telephone: 1 800 228 1966
Fax: 208 265 2488
e-mail: info@thorne.com
www.thorne.com

How to Learn More About Nutrition

The Institute for Optimum Nutrition (ION) is a London-based leading charity within its field, devoted to promoting health and well-being through nutrition by providing seminars and workshops, foundation courses, a three-year nutrition consultants' diploma course, membership scheme, *Optimum Nutrition* magazine, library and information service plus a nutrition clinic. For enquiries or a free information pack call the Help Desk on: 44 (0) 20 8877 9993 or e-mail info@ion.ac.uk

I.O.N.
Blades Court
Deodar Road
London SW15 2NU
UK

How to Find a Qualified Nutritionist

Contact the Institute for Optimum Nutrition (details above) for a register of qualified practitioners. You can also obtain a register of practitioners from the British Association of Nutritional Therapists at BCM BANT, London, WC1N 3XX.
Telephone/Fax: 44 (0) 870 606 1284.

About the Author

Erica White, Dip.ION, qualified with excellence after three years of training at the Institute for Optimum Nutrition and is a member of the British Association of Nutritional Therapists. She is Director of **Nutritionhelp Ltd** and members of her team are available for personal nutritional consultations and also for postal consultations worldwide. Clients are provided with a detailed questionnaire from which their nutritional status may be assessed and they then receive a full report with findings and recommendations which is either discussed at a personal consultation or sent with an explanatory covering letter to postal clients. This is followed by three months of 'back-up' contact as needed (by telephone or e-mail) within the price of the consultation to enable ongoing support. A review analysis is strongly recommended at three-monthly intervals so that the situation may be monitored and recommendations adjusted as progress is made. Fees on request.

Telephone: 44 (0) 1702 472085
Fax: 44 (0) 1702 471935
e-mail: reception@nutritionhelp.com
Website: http://www.nutritionhelp.com

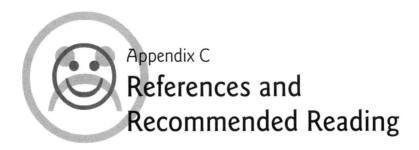

Appendix C

References and Recommended Reading

Ballweg, Mary Lou. 'Endometriosis and Candidiasis: More startling connections', in *Overcoming Endometriosis*, Arlington Books, 1988.

Bland, Jeffrey. 'Hidden Diseases Caused by Candida', in *Preventive Medicine*, 3 (4): 12, 1984.

Bredell, Frank. *The Spores that Attack You: When Your Immune System Can't Protect You*, Felmore Limited Health Publications, Tunbridge Wells (undated).

Brostoff, Jonathan and Gamlin, Linda. *Food Allergy and Intolerance*, Bloomsbury, 1989.

Chaitow, Leon. *Beat Fatigue Workbook*, Thorsons, 1988.

Chaitow, Leon. *Candida albicans: Could Yeast be Your Problem?*, Thorsons, 1985.

Chaitow, Leon. *Post Viral Fatigue Syndrome*, Dent, London, 1989.

Colby, Jane. 'M.E.: A polio by another name', in *What Doctors Don't Tell You*, 6:9, December 1995.

Crook, William G. *The Yeast Connection: A Medical Breakthrough*, 2nd ed., Professional Books, Jackson, Tennessee, 1984.

Davies, Stephen and Stewart, Alan. *Nutritional Medicine*, Pan Books, London, 1987.

Davis, Adelle. *Let's Get Well*, Unwin Paperbacks, London, 1985.

Golan, Ralph, MD. *Optimal Wellness*, Ballantine Books, New York, 1995.

Hale, Teresa. *Breathing Free*, Hodder & Stoughton, 1999.

Holford, Patrick. *The Optimum Nutrition Bible*, Piatkus, 1997.

Holford, Patrick. *100% Health*, Piatkus, 1998.

Jacobs, Gill. *Beat Candida Through Diet*, Vermillion, 1997.

Jones, Doris. 'How vaccines can cause M.E.' in *What Doctors Don't Tell You*, 6:9, December 1995.

Langer, S.E. and Scheer, J.F. *Solved – The Riddle of Illness*, Keats Publishing, New Canaan, Connecticut, 1984.

Lipski, Elizabeth. *Digestive Wellness*, Keats, 1996.

McWhirter, Jane. *The Practical Guide to Candida*, All Hallows House Foundation, 1995.

Odds, F.C. *Candida and Candidosis*, Bailliere Tindall, London, 1988.

Pauling, Linus. 'The Last Interview', in *Optimum Nutrition*, 7:2, Winter 1994.

Sears, Barry. *The Zone*, Regan Books, Harper Collins, 1995.

Shaw, William. *Biological Treatments for Autism and PDD*, Health, USA, 1998. (Available from The Great Plains laboratory – see address in Appendix B.)

Stalmatski, Alexander. *Freedom from Asthma*, Kyle Cathie, 1997.

Stevens, Laura J. 'Endometriosis and Yeast: A New Connection', in *Overcoming Endometriosis*, Arlington Books, 1988.

The Vaccination Bible, What Doctors Don't Tell You, The Wallace Press, 2000.

Other books by Erica White:

Candida-kuren, published in Norwegian, Ex Libris, Oslo, 1998.

Beat Candida Cookbook, Thorsons, 1999.

'Candidiasis – An Update', *Lamberts Bulletin*, Lamberts Healthcare Ltd., Tunbridge Wells, 1999.

Doughnuts & Temples, Monarch Books, 2000.

Index

abattoirs 34
abdominal cramps 22
accidents 63
acidophilus *see also* probiotics 132
addictions 26–7, 43, 57, 59, 88, 223
additives 35, 47, 49, 92, 222
addresses 241–5
adolescents 15
Adrenal Stress Index 71
adrenals 62, 64–72, 89–90, 93
advertising 35
ageing process 29
AIDS 39
air conditioning 49
alarm response 65
alcohol 26, 29, 50, 57, 59
    four-point plan 113
    guidelines 223
    low blood sugar 90, 92
    stress 66
allergies 6, 12, 21–32, 39, 50
    candida 98
    eczema 100

environment 129
gut dysbiosis 107–8
stress 62–4
aloe vera 118–19
aluminium 46, 47
Alzheimer's Disease 46
amalgam fillings 43, 46–7, 116, 127
American pancakes 210
amino acids 31–2, 37
    diet 113
    slow progress 128
    stress 69
    thyroid 86
    toxicity 50, 52
amylase 26
anaemia 83
anaphylactic shock 21, 22
animals 30
anti-inflammatories 29
antibiotics 6, 23, 35, 39
    antifungals 118
    babies 104
    candida 99
    gut dysbiosis 95–6, 107

probiotics 120
antibodies 17, 19, 50
   candida 102
   gut dysbiosis 105
   stress 69
antidepressants 73
antifungals 96, 100, 116–20
   die-off 124–5
   four-point plan 111
   way ahead 131–2
antioxidants 38, 50
anxiety 5, 6, 8, 63
   die-off 126
   gut dysbiosis 106
   low blood sugar 87
   stress 64, 65
   supplements 70
artificial sweeteners 89, 222
aspirin 29
asthma 21–5, 31–2, 48, 77–8, 100
athletes 45
attitude 232
atypical polio 2, 16
aubergine quiche 205–6
avocado dessert 213–14

babies 103–4
baked beans 196
baked chips 207–8
baked egg custard 212
baked lemon chicken breasts 208
barley 26
Barnes, B. 83, 84
bean and vegetable stew 203–4
beans 37, 71, 90–1
bee-stings 21
beliefs 227–37
bereavement 63

bile 54, 125
biochemical individuality 114–15
BioMed International 55, 242
blackcurrant tea loaf 216–17
Bland, J. 51
bloating 5, 22, 101, 104
blood pressure 70, 81
blood sugar 71, 87–93, 223
blood tests 83, 105
blurred vision 75
bowel diseases 29, 37, 98
brain scans 16
breakfast recipes 192–5
breast-feeding 25, 100, 102
breathing techniques 32, 48, 76–9
British Medical Association 46
bromelain 26
bronchodilators 32, 77
Brostoff, J. 21
buggies 47
bulimia 27
burns 29
Buteyko, K. 77, 78

cabagin 70
cadmium 46, 47
caffeine 93, 137, 223
calcium 43, 44, 54, 72
cancer 50
candida 28–30, 32, 41, 52
   antifungals 118
   die-off 123
   four-point plan 111–22
   gut dysbiosis 94–5, 105–7
   hyperventilation 79
   low blood sugar 92
   parasites 96–8
   score sheet 238–40
   symptoms 131
candidiasis 7, 94, 101, 126

caprylic acid 100, 116–17, 119, 124–5
carbohydrates 37, 70–1
    four-point plan 112
    guidelines 220
    low blood sugar 90–2
carbon monoxide 49
carob cake 217–18
carob crunchies 215
Carroll, L. 21
carrot cake 214
case studies 138–79
Cathcart, R. 39
causes 11–12
chain of events 6
Chaitow, L. 20, 39, 94
cheese 36
chemicals 33, 47, 92, 129
chicken 90–2
chicken burgers 200–1
chicken pox 15
chicken risotto 204–5
chickweed 119
children 45–6, 48–9
chocolate 8, 26–7, 36
    lifestyle 59
    low blood sugar 88, 90, 93
choices 232
cholesterol 38
Christianity 228–37
chromium 56, 90, 93
Chronic Fatigue Immune
    Dysfunction Association
    (CFIDS) 1–2
Chronic Fatigue Syndrome
    (CFS) 1–12
cigarettes 43, 46, 50, 64, 66
Circadian rhythm 66
coeliac disease 28–9
coffee 8, 26–7, 36, 40
    four-point plan 112

    guidelines 223
    lifestyle 56–6, 59
    low blood sugar 88, 90, 93
    stress 64, 66
    substitutes 54
Colby, J. 16, 17–18
colds 18, 67, 79
colic 103
colitis 29
colon 101
Comprehensive Digestive Stool
    Analysis (CDSA) 95
Comprehensive Parasitology 95
concentration 5, 6, 74, 78, 106
constipation 5, 51, 54, 101, 103, 129
contraception see also Pill 32
corn cakes 217
cortisol 66–70
cottage cheese 71, 90–2
cow's milk 25, 26
Coxsachie 15–17, 19
crab 22
creamy carob dessert 209
Crohn's disease 29
Crook, W. 106
crudités 198
crunchy cereal 193
crying 5
cystitis 5, 6, 101
Cytomegalovirus 15

dairy produce 22, 26, 99, 120
dandelion coffee 125, 128, 223
Darwin, C. 2
Davies, S. 64
daylight 49
death 232
dentures 119
depression 5–6, 22, 37
    die-off 126

gut dysbiosis 106
low blood sugar 87–8
stress 63–4, 71, 73
supplements 70
thyroid 83
dessert recipes 208–18
detergents 29, 30
detoxification 52–3, 125
dextrose 112
DHEA 66–9
diabetes 36, 56, 81, 87–8
Diagnos-Techs 68, 81, 242
diarrhoea 5, 22, 31, 39
gut dysbiosis 101, 103
thyroid 82
die-off 71, 117, 120, 123–6, 131
diesel 31
diet 6, 31, 36, 38–9
anti-candida 183–8
deficiencies 44
die-off 124
four-point plan 111, 112–14
guidelines 219–23
lifestyle 56, 59
low blood sugar 89
motivation 132
questionnaires 115
slow progress 129–30
toxicity 54
digestion 26, 28–9, 43, 118, 127
dinner parties 113
dinner recipes 202–8
diverticulitis 37
dizziness 5, 78, 87–8
doctors 4, 32, 69, 96, 100–1
drugs 49–50, 57, 59
antifungals 117–118
gut dysbiosis 99
thyroid 83

eating habits 7–8, 56–7, 219,
233–4
eczema 22–5, 32, 48
anti-fungals 119
babies 104
steroids 100
eggplant quiche 205–6
eggs 71
embroidery 58
emulsification 35
endometriosis 103
endoscopy 105
energy levels 89
enterovirus 17
environment 30–1, 35–6, 42
breast-feeding 100
free radicals 50
slow progress 128–9
stress 63
toxicity 47
environmental factors 22
enzymes 26, 29, 43, 81, 120, 127
Epstein-Barr virus 15, 17, 19
essential fatty acids 29, 37, 40,
44, 115, 222
Evening Primrose Oil 44
exercise 8–9, 53–4, 58–60
faith 231
low blood sugar 93
stress 71
exhaustion 5, 9, 49, 57, 67, 78,
87

faith 227–37
falafel 199
farmers 48
fatigue 87
fats 36, 40, 72
fear 8–10, 64–5
Feldman, D. 102
fertilizers 35

fibre 37, 51
First World War 35
fish 37, 72, 90, 92, 221
fish cakes 193–4
fish oil 44
flax 44, 51
flu *see* influenza
fluid retention 114
folic acid 38, 44
food 8, 33, 36, 38–9
    avoiding 183–5
    diaries 27
    enjoying 186–8
    organic 54
    toxicity 50
four-point plan 111–22, 124, 131
free radicals 38, 50, 53
fructose 34, 89, 92, 112
fruit 34, 50, 70, 89, 92, 112
fumes 30–1, 46, 49, 108

garlic 118
gas 30–1, 49, 108, 129
German measles 15
giddiness 75
ginger cake 215
glandular fever 15, 107
glucose 37, 87–93, 99, 112
Glucose Tolerance Factor (GTF)
    90, 93
glue 30
gluten 26, 28, 95, 191
Golan, R. 104
grains 26, 33, 36, 50
    four-point plan 112
    low blood sugar 89–92
    stress 70–1
Great Plains Laboratory 105, 242
Great Smokies Diagnostic
    Laboratory 28, 52, 55, 95,
    241

grins 34
gut dysbiosis 12, 94–108
gut flora 19, 23–4, 94, 113, 120
gut virus 17

hair mineral analysis 47, 55
Hale, T. 32, 77–8, 79
hayfever 21–2, 31, 79
headaches 5, 22, 27, 53
    hyperventilation 75
    lifestyle 57
    low blood sugar 87–8
health 234–6
Health Interlink 28, 52, 95, 105,
    241
heart diseases 35–6, 50
Helpers 38
hepatitis 39
herbs 117–18
herpes 15
Herxheimer's reaction 123
hives 23
hobbies 58–9, 74
Holford, P. 31, 39–40, 44–5, 115
honey 34, 89
hormones 24, 35, 37, 62
    candida 101–3
    faith 228
    gut dysbiosis 98
    stress 66, 68, 71–2
    thyroid 81, 82–3
hot flushes 37
house-plants 30
HRT 6, 24, 32, 99, 116
hummus 197
hydrochloric acid 127–8
hydrogenation 35
hyperactivity 23
hyperventilation 12, 75–80
hypochondria 4
hypoglycaemia 12, 56, 87–93, 94

hypothalamus 66
hysterectomies 24

Iceland Disease 2
identity crises 10
immune system 5–6, 7, 11
    allergies 22–7, 30
    babies 104
    candida 97–8
    four-point plan 114
    gut dysbiosis 107
    low blood sugar 87
    nutrition 38
    nutritional deficiencies 40–3
    progress 128
    steroids 116
    stress 63–4, 69, 72
    toxicity 46–8, 50–1
    viral infections 15–16, 18–20
immunization 24–5
Industrial Revolution 33
infections 39, 83, 94, 99, 107
influenza 15, 18–19, 67, 79
inhalers 24, 32, 48, 77
insomnia 6, 57, 71
Institute of Optimum Nutrition
    (ION) 40–1, 108, 114,
    244–5
insulin 88–90
interferon 18
Intestinal Permeability Test 24,
    95
intestines 6–7, 12, 15
    allergies 22–3, 26, 28–9
    breast-feeding 100
    gut dysbiosis 101, 103, 107
    parasites 95–6
    probiotics 120
    stress 69, 70
intolerances 21–2, 28, 95
    progress 127

recipes 191
    stress 64
iodine 84, 85
iron 38
irritability 5–6, 23, 27, 49
    gut dysbiosis 106
    low blood sugar 88
irritable bowels 5, 101

joints 5, 23, 67, 83
    arthritic 101
    candida 98

kedgeree 201
Kent, Duchess of 2
kidneys 49, 101

L-Glutamine 113
lactase 26
lactic acid 60, 120–1
lactose 41, 54, 73, 112, 120
lactulose 29
Langer, S. 82, 84
lead 46, 47
leaky gut syndrome 24, 26, 28–9,
    32, 50, 95, 106
learning difficulties 46
lemon and carrot crumble
    212–13
lemon cheesecake 209–10
lemon and coconut sauce 211
lentil wedges 200
lifestyle 7, 12, 36, 56–61, 72, 231
linseed 51, 54, 72
linseed oil 44
lipase 26
Lipski, E. 100
liquorice 68, 69–70
liver 6, 30, 32, 49–51
    die-off 125
    low blood sugar 90, 93

stress 65
 toxicity 52–3, 55
local anaesthetics 31, 108
low blood sugar 12, 36, 87–93,
 94, 220
lunch recipes 197–201
lycopene 50
lymphatic system 9, 53, 58, 60,
 71

macronutrients 37
malingering 4
malnutrition 33
malt 112
mannitol 29
margarine 35
marigold 119
ME 18, 20, 94
meals 90–2
meat 34–5, 99
memory 5–6, 78, 106
menopause 32, 37, 43, 45
 antifungals 116
 faith 230
 gut dysbiosis 99
menstruation 81, 85, 102, 227
menus 112, 189–90
mercury 43, 46–7, 116, 127
metals 46
micronutrients 37
migraines 6, 36
milk thistle 55
minerals 31, 33, 36–42
 action plan 44
 die-off 124
 four-point plan 115–16
 lifestyle 56
 low blood sugar 90, 93
 toxicity 47, 50, 54
money 229–30
mononucleosis 15

mood swings 5, 6
mould 30, 112, 128
muesli base 192–3
Multiple Sclerosis 47
muscles 5, 9, 15, 18, 23
 candida 98
 gut dysbiosis 101
 hyperventilation 75, 78
 lifestyle 60
 stress 67
 thyroid 83
 toxicity 53
music 57
Myalgic Encephalomyelitis (ME)
 1–2
mycelia 98

nappy rash 103
National Health Service 229
National Hospital for Nervous
 Diseases 23
nausea 5, 9, 53, 75, 101
nicotine 57, 59
Nightingale, F. 2
non-paralytic polio 16
North Sea gas 23, 31
nutrition 235
 deficiencies 12, 29, 33–45
 status 19–20
nutritional supplements 7, 29,
 31–2, 41–4, 70
 four-point plan 111, 114–16
 low blood sugar 93
 suppliers 243–4
 thyroid 84–5
nutritionists 8, 26, 29, 31–2
 contacts 245
 deficiencies 40, 44
 liver 52
 parasites 95
 stress 70, 72

support 121
thyroid 84
toxicity 55
nuts 50, 72, 91

oatcakes 195
oatmeal porridge 192
oats 26, 92
Odds, F.C. 101, 106
oils 37, 45, 221
osteoporosis 43, 100

paint 30–1
painting 58
palpitations 5, 75
pancreas 88–90
panic 5–6, 23, 75–6, 79, 87–8
papain 26
paper bags 76
parasites 29, 95–7, 117, 129
Pauling, L. 39
peanuts 21, 22
pease pudding slices 195
perfumes 30, 108
pesticides 30, 35, 48–9
petrol 30, 36, 108
pharmaceuticals 47, 83, 95, 117
Phase I detoxification 52
Phase II detoxification 52–3
Pill 6, 24, 32, 73, 99, 103
piperade 202–3
pituitary 66
pizza scones 198–9
plastics 30
poisson del mar 206–7
polio 16, 18
politics 36
pollen 23, 30, 31
pollution 12, 25, 30, 33
    breast-feeding 100
    deficiencies 35, 42

stress 63
toxicity 46–55
polyunsaturates 35
Post-Viral Fatigue Syndrome 2
potato and parsnip bake 207
poultry 37, 221
prayer 10, 74, 235
pregnancy 45, 47, 102, 103
premenstrual tension (PMT) 5,
    37, 40, 103, 104
preservatives 35, 47, 92, 222
probiotics 111, 120–1
profits 35
progress 127–30
propolis 118–19
prostoglandins 222
protein 37, 70–1, 90–2, 220–2
psychological stress 63
pulse tests 27–8
pulses 37, 71, 90

questionnaires 115, 131,
    238–40

radiation 29
recipes 191–218
Recommended Daily Allowance
    (RDA) 42
redundancy 63
Reference Nutrient Intake (RNI)
    42
refined foods 29, 33–4, 36
    diet 112
    low blood sugar 89, 92
    stress 70
    toxicity 50
relapses 53
relaxation 57–9, 65, 74, 231
rennin 26
research 3, 4
rest 57, 59, 67

rhinitis 32
Royal Free Disease 1
Royal Free Hospital 1
rubella 15
rye 26, 71
rye slice 216

St John's Wort 70, 73
salads 220
saliva testing 52, 67
salt 222
scrambled eggs 194
Sears, B. 71, 91
seaweed 84–5
seeds 45, 50, 72, 91
selenium 38, 43–4, 47, 50, 54
senile dementia 46
sensitivities 21–2, 25–6, 28–30,
    96
Shaw, W. 105
shelf-life 34
shivering 5
shopping 231
Siberian ginseng 69, 73
sick building syndrome 49
silymarin 55
sinusitis 23, 32
sleep 57, 59, 66–7, 78
snacks 90–2
soaps 30
social stress 63
soda bread rolls 197
spices 29
Stalmatski, A. 23, 77–8
star rating 112–13, 191
starch 26
starvation 29
steamed pudding 211–12
steroids 6, 24, 32, 48
    asthma 100
    babies 104

candida 102
gut dysbiosis 99
hyperventilation 77
immune system 116
Stewart, A. 64
stool culture 104
stool testing 95–7, 117
stress 8, 11–12, 19–20, 62–74
    breathing techniques 79
    lifestyle 58
    low blood sugar 93
    slow progress 129
Stuttaford, T. 17
sucrose 34, 40, 89, 112
sugar 6, 34, 36, 40
    blood 87–93
    candida 98–9
    four-point plan 112–13
    guidelines 220
    lifestyle 56
    stress 65, 73
    toxicity 54
sulphur 50, 53
suppliers 243–4
support 4, 121–2, 124
Suppressors 38
surgery 29
sweating 5
Sweden 47
sweet tooth 34, 113
symptoms 4–5, 9, 11
    allergens 107
    allergies 22, 24, 26, 29
    amalgam fillings 47
    candida 131–2
    candidiasis 94
    die-off 123, 125
    gut dysbiosis 104, 106
    hyperventilation 75–6, 79
    low blood sugar 87, 88
    nutritional deficiencies 41

questionnaires 40, 115
thyroid activity 82, 84
synthetic materials 49

T cells 38
tea 8, 26–7, 40
    four-point plan 112
    guidelines 223
    lifestyle 56–7, 59
    low blood sugar 88, 90, 93
    stress 64, 66
tea tree oil 119, 121
temperature test 83, 84–5, 86
temptations 236
Third World 36
thrush 5–6, 103, 119, 121, 133
thyroid 12, 19, 67, 81–6
tofu 90, 92
tomato and tuna topping 202
toxins 9, 12, 24, 30, 32
    breast-feeding 100
    die-off 124, 125–6
    gut dysbiosis 98, 106
    lifestyle 58, 60
    pollution 46–55
    pregnancy 102
trans fatty acids 35
trauma 29, 63

University of Wales 121
urine testing 28–9, 52, 105, 128

vaccinations 15–17, 25
Valerian 70
varnish 30, 31
vegetables 36, 50, 70–1, 90–2
veggie pie 203
viral infections 11–12, 15–20, 39, 99

virus 7
vitamins 29, 31, 33, 37–9
    action plan 44
    antioxidants 50
    deficiencies 41–3
    die-off 124
    four-point plan 115–16
    low blood sugar 90, 93
    stress 70, 72–3
    thyroid 83
    toxicity 47, 51, 54

water 51, 54, 125, 222
water retention 5
website 246
weight-loss 28, 113–14
wheat 22, 26–7, 71, 92
wholefoods 31
wind 5, 101, 104
withdrawal symptoms 26
work routines 73–4
workaholics 57

yeast 30, 41, 73, 79
    anti-fungals 118
    candida 98, 102
    diet 112
    four-point plan 112, 114
    gut dysbiosis 94, 97, 101, 105, 106
    infections 6–7
yoghurt 37, 90–1, 120
yoghurt soda bread 196–7
yoghurt surprise 208
Yuppie flu 2, 57

zinc 29, 43–4, 54, 90